Encyclopedia of Little Known Secrets of Perfect Natural Health

By Frank W. Cawood and Janice McCall Failes

Acknowledgments

Healing is a special process that requires love and concern This book is also the result of the concern, love and talent of many people.

To all the staff members who contributed their treasured healing secrets: Jo Bauer, Linda Gunnan, Anne Joyner, Barbara McMillan, Lois Parker, Linda Sciullo Marcia Ulery, and Debbie Williams.

To Linda Sciullo, for your conscientious proofreading and forgiving patience.

To Betty Whitfield, for your superb editing and thoughtful suggestions.

To Debbie Williams, for your art work and design.

To all the staff of FC&A, for your support and willingness to help.

To our spouses, Gayle and B., for your constant encouragement and abiding love.

But, most of all, our thanks and praise is for our Lord and Savior, Jesus Christ, who as one with the Heavenly Father created us, heals us and gives us eternal life, through the power of His Holy Spirit.

Dedicated to Jesus Christ
— the greatest healer of all time.

Beloved, I pray that in all respects you may prosper
and be in good health.
— 3 John: 2

'For I will restore you to health.
And I will heal you of your wounds,'
declares the Lord.
— Jeremiah 30:15

Quotations from
The New American Standard Bible

Table of Contents

Introduction

We are all going to have health problems of one sort or another, but have you ever wondered why some people are almost never sick? Why they seem to be in almost super perfect health? Many of these healthy people understand and practice natural remedies that keep them feeling good.

Staying in good health may be overcoming something that seems small, like a sore throat or tiredness... or it may be preventing something which threatens your overall health, like heart disease or maturity onset diabetes. This new book, *Encyclopedia of Little Known Secrets of Perfect Natural Health*, reveals hundreds of tips to help you stay healthy.

In addition to natural remedies, the book sometimes mentions certain medical treatments. Medical treatment should not be ignored, but natural prevention or treatment may help too.

The natural healing secrets and health tips reported in this book are not guaranteed to succeed with everyone. As we wrote this book, we realized that we could not pass judgement on the effectiveness of most health secrets that we discovered. Some of these secrets may work for you but not for other people. Some may work for other people but not for you. Many of the health secrets reported in this book may be controversial or unproven by controlled scientific studies. We have reported the ideas in this book simply because there is some evidence that they have worked for some people. In doing this, we have attempted to separate fact from fiction and to give special attention to remedies which have been confirmed by scientific research. We have attempted, wherever possible, to verify the accuracy of information reported in this book. Nevertheless, since these are only reports of the research or ideas of other people, we cannot guarantee their safety or effectiveness.

Because of the possibility of errors in reporting the research of others, and because medical science is such a rapidly expanding field with new developments reported each day, we ask that you consult carefully with your own physician before trying any of the health tips listed in this book.

It can be dangerous to rely on self-treatment or home remedies and neglect proven medical treatments, such as surgery in cases of cancer. A good physician is the best judge of what type of medical treatment may be needed for certain diseases. It's good to choose a physician who is open-minded about safe, natural methods of prevention and treatment.

Allergy Relief — Airborne Allergens

• Here are some common allergens (things that trigger allergic symptoms):
> dusts, molds, and pollens
> animal hair or feathers
> strong odors
> petroleum-based gases and fumes or dust associated with coal heat
> insecticides
> hair sprays
> perfumes
> waxes and polishes
> detergents and bleach
> room deodorizers
> gasoline
> paint and paint thinners
> tar
> plastics
> lubricants
> asphalt and cement
> cigarette, cigar and pipe smoke
> Inhaled insect parts frequently cause allergic reactions. Hairs, scales or other body parts of insects like houseflies, mayflies, moths, cockroaches, spiders, honeybees, caddis flies, locusts and mites may cause problems.

• Many people have seasonal allergies, like an allergy to pollen or mold. Some of these allergies are nicknamed "hay fever", but the name is not accurate. It isn't hay, but pollen, that causes the problem, and the problem isn't a fever but an allergic reaction!

The pollen season begins in February in the southern United States, but starts later the farther north you travel. "Pollen counts", which measure the amount of pollen in the air in a 24-hour period, are available on many TV weather programs to help you. According to the American Academy of Allergy and Immunology, a count of 50 or more is considered high, 30-50 is moderate, and 10-20 is a low count. During the heavy pollen season in your area, or a day with a high pollen count, you should avoid going outside or opening your windows.

• Sneezing, runny nose, nasal congestion, shortness of breath, sore throat, watery eyes, itchy eyes or wheezing are the most common allergic reactions to airborne particles.

The best way to relieve allergy symptoms is to avoid the allergen if it is known. Be aware which seasons of the year are the times when your allergy flares up, and take special precautions during those times. To guard against aggravating your allergy to airborne things:

> Mow the lawn regularly to help lower grass pollen.

> Cut all weeds as soon as possible.

> Use air-conditioning in your house. Central air-conditioning helps control airborne allergens. A window air-conditioner is recommended for the bedroom of the allergy sufferer.

> Use air filters (electrostatic air filters if possible).

> Change vacuum cleaner filters. A central vacuum cleaning system is best because the system won't exhaust air and dust into the living area. If you don't have a central system, be sure to keep the windows open when vacuuming.

> Radiant heat is best for allergy sufferers. Forced air heat circulates dust and causes the house to dry out.

> Keep your office and home as clean as possible, especially bedrooms.

> Avoid housecleaning while the allergy suffering person is present.

> Use non-allergenic covers on mattresses and pillows.

> Use polyester or other non-allergenic pillows, and replace them at least every three years.

> Vacuum fabric-covered furniture frequently.

> Don't keep houseplants that have a strong fragrance or plants that require a lot of water because they could mildew.

> Use an artificial Christmas tree to reduce the possibility of mold and mildew.

> Have washable curtains and avoid heavy draperies.

> Don't hang wet clothes or linens outside to dry. Use a dryer and keep the filter clean.

> Don't use rugs, carpets, stuffed toys, furry toys, quilts or afghans in the bedroom.

> Don't use strong-smelling cleaners, polishes, moth balls, perfume or chemicals in the bedroom.

> Don't use aerosol sprays of any kind.

> Store books in boxes or warm, dry areas. Get rid of old books which may have mildewed.

> Sterilize the air ducts at the beginning of each cold season. Clean the air ducts and filters regularly.

> Keep household pets out of bedrooms or out of the house if possible.

> Don't allow cigarettes, pipes or cigars to be smoked in or around the house.

> Avoid using wallpaper in the bedrooms.

> Keep physically fit and exercise regularly. Congestion in the nose may be worse when you are resting or sitting still than when you are active. Exercise can be as simple as swimming, walking or bike riding. Exercising indoors may protect you from allergens in the outside air.

> Maintain good general health.

> Avoid breathing fine powders like talcum powder, dusting powder or powdered artificial

sweeteners like Equal® or Sweet 'n Low®. They can irritate the breathing system.

> Avoid using nasal drops or sprays. If they are overused, nasal sprays can actually cause allergy symptoms to return.

> Keep the windows and vents of your car closed when driving. Use air-conditioning in your car.

> Avoid early morning activity. According to the American Academy of Allergies, pollen is heaviest in the air before 10:00 a.m.

> Avoid extreme temperature changes. Follow the weather forecast so you can avoid strong winds, drastic changes in humidity, barometric pressure or temperature.

> A report in the medical journal, Lancet (1:1079), says that fungus spores and small particles of pollen may stay in the air after a large storm. The Lancet report recommends that asthmatics and people with allergies to airborne particles stay indoors for a day after a heavy storm.

> Consider taking a long vacation. Sometimes a long vacation is enough to help relieve severe allergic reactions. Plan your vacation during the peak of the season when your allergy flares up. If possible, go where you won't be affected by your allergen.

• If you take antihistamines for your allergies, drink plenty of fluids to avoid tooth decay.

Antihistamines dry up the saliva in the mouth and nasal passages. The decrease in saliva can cause an increase in the number of cavities and gum problems, according to an article in Family Circle (7/8/86). People taking antihistamines have more risk of tooth decay. If you are on antihistamines, brush your teeth more often and drink more water or other sugar-free drinks to avoid an increase in dental problems.

• If your allergic reactions are severe, you may want to consider moving to a less-populated and less-polluted area. Be careful to take an extended visit to an area before making a complete move there. Some areas may be great for certain allergy sufferers but not for you. Many allergy sufferers will develop a new allergy once they have lived in a community for a while. Do not rush into a permanent move.

If you must live in a big city, try to avoid congested areas with heavy traffic because cars and trucks create noxious exhaust fumes. Avoid areas with known industrial pollution.

Also see: **Asthma.**

Allergy Relief — Allergies to Cosmetics

Cosmetics include make-up and the many products both sexes use to clean, condition and "beautify" hair and bodies. Allergic reactions are quite common to these cosmetics: deodorants, soap, perfume, cologne, shaving cream, after-shave lotion, shampoo, mouthwash, lipstick, eyeliner, mascara, eye shadow, blush, foundation, hair dye, hair bleach, hair coloring, hair spray, hair mousse, skin cleanser, hair remover, suntan lotion, tanning cream, nail polish, nail polish remover and the glue on artificial nails.

Localized allergic reactions to these products may cause skin rash, dryness or irritation. General allergic reactions can affect the whole body by causing hives, congestion, asthma or swelling. Many allergic reactions to cosmetics can cause premature aging of the skin if it becomes damaged. The most commonly occurring reaction to cosmetics is skin dermatitis, with symptoms like irritation, redness, itching, swelling, rash, scaling, blisters and dryness.

People often wonder why they suddenly react to a product that they have been using for several years, perhaps throughout their whole lives. But many times people reach a sensitivity point — that means that the body may be able to tolerate the cosmetic in small doses, but the body eventually reaches its tolerance level, and an allergic reaction occurs.

Some women discover allergies while they are pregnant. Many of these allergies will disappear after the birth of the child. However, some women with severe allergies have experienced the opposite effect — their allergies have cleared up during their pregnancies!

The best method of treating cosmetic allergies is to avoid the offending cosmetics. However, until you know which cosmetics are causing the problem, here are some suggestions to help keep the reactions from becoming unbearable:

• Keep your body, hair and clothes as clean as possible. Avoid touching your face or eyes with your hands. For example, if you rub your eyes, hand lotion may irritate them.

• If you think you know what product you are allergic to, try switching to a different brand. Sometimes the allergen may be an ingredient that only one manufacturer uses. However, changing products is recommended only if the initial allergic reaction was not severe.

• Consider and evaluate the ingredients before purchasing a cosmetic product. Unfortunately, to protect secret formulas, federal regulations allow some ingredients to be listed in very general categories. This may make it difficult to determine if the cosmetic you select contains the offending allergen.

• If you are taking a prescription drug, check with your doctor to make sure the reaction is not a known side effect or a photosensitive reaction of your medicine. "Photosensitive reactions" occur when you're exposed to sunlight while taking a prescribed drug.

• Try switching to hypoallergenic cosmetics. However, according to the Allergy Foundation of America, not all hypoallergenic cosmetics meet their manufacturer's claims. For a complete and up-to-date list of the products that are best, you can write directly to The Asthma and Allergy Foundation — see their address in our *Appendix One: Special Agencies to Consult.*

• If you discover that you can use certain cosmetics, try to keep your applicators very clean. Your allergies may be a reaction to make-up applicators like sponges, brushes, eye wands and puffs. Keeping them very clean or trying new ways to apply your make-up may help relieve the allergy.

• If truly hypoallergenic products don't eliminate the reactions, stop using ALL make-up and cosmetics. After about six months of being completely allergy-free, you can try re-introducing some cosmetics, one at a time if your reactions were not too serious or life-threatening. You may discover that you can use some products but not others.

• Use a bland, unscented soap to wash your face, skin and hair. Using the soap on your hair will help wash away any remains of your previous shampoo and conditioner.

• Try to stop using any lotions or creams like hand lotion, baby oil, cleansing cream or moisturizers. When showering or bathing, use warm water, not hot. Hot water dries out your skin, making it more sensitive.

• Avoid using nail polish. Nail polish can cause allergic reactions in many places, not just on your hands. Nail polish can irritate eyes or facial skin, since we touch our eyes and face with our fingers and hands. Even a man can experience an allergic reaction to a woman's nail polish or other cosmetics if he is in close contact with her!

• Discuss your allergies and concerns with your hair-dresser. You may discover that one of their products is causing your allergic reaction. If they don't have alternative products, or won't serve you with little or no cosmetics, find another beauty or barber shop. Also, if you plan to have your hair tinted, colored or permed, insist on a skin test before the full treatment. A small skin test and a little patience can prevent a severe reaction later.

Alzheimer's Disease

• According to Dr. Robert Friedland of the National Institute on Aging, Alzheimer's disease attacks the brain cells. It usually affects senior citizens. Alzheimer's victims can live as long as ten years, but death normally occurs within a few months of the onset of symptoms. Loss of memory, depression, changes in personality, wandering, delusions, loss of bladder and bowel control, loss of ability to talk and a reduction in the ability to complete the everyday tasks of living are signs of Alzheimer's disease.

• Memory loss in Alzheimer's patients is different than memory loss in other adults. Lisa P. Gwyther, who wrote the book, Care of Alzheimer's Patients: A Manual for Nursing Home Staff, explains that many adults forget things. A normal adult will forget part of the event but the Alzheimer's victim will forget the whole event, says Gwyther. A normal adult will eventually remember what they forgot. They will feel guilty because they forgot something. A person with Alzheimer's will forget the event, never remember it in the future, and won't even realize that they have forgotten anything, she explains. It won't be important to them. Their memories also continue to get worse, according to Gwyther.

• Low levels of vitamin B12 (cobalamin) and zinc were found in people with Alzheimer's disease in a study published in the Journal of Orthomolecular Psychiatry. The research conducted in The Netherlands showed that if Alzheimer's is recognized at an early stage, treatment with vitamin B12 and zinc may help restore memory. Liver, meat, milk, dairy products, fish and eggs are good sources of vitamin B12. Zinc is found naturally in liver, seafood, dairy products, meat, eggs and whole-grain products.

• Loss of estrogen may play a part in the development of Alzheimer's in postmenopausal women, according to Dr. Bruce McEwen of Rockefeller University. Dr. McEwen found that women with Alzheimer's had lower estrogen levels than their healthy counterparts, reports an article in the Saturday Evening Post (258:9). He also discovered that estrogen, a natural hormone, seems to have a reaction on the brain cells that is opposite to the reaction from Alzheimer's disease. Alzheimer's disease causes nerve cells to degenerate, while estrogen causes them to thrive. Initial tests are being conducted on the use of estrogen in female Alzheimer's patients. The final role of estrogen supplements in treating Alzheimer's victims is not known.

• Dr. Daniel Peter Perl from the Mount Sinai Hospital in New York suggests that acid rain "leeches aluminum out of the soil into our drinking water". Since autopsies of Alzheimer's victims have revealed higher than normal levels of aluminum in the brain tissue, researchers are evaluating the role of aluminum in the development of the disease (<u>New</u> <u>England</u> <u>Journal</u> <u>of</u> <u>Medicine</u> 1980). Dr. Perl believes that acid rain may be dangerously increasing our exposure to aluminum.

Angina

• Men suffering from angina pectoris, pain in the chest associated with heart disease, should try wearing a girdle around the waist, according to Dr. Peter J. Steincrohn. This doctor believes, and has supporting testimonies, that wearing a girdle (often called an abdominal support) helps ease the strain on the heart. Supporting the abdominal muscles helps increase circulation. To ask a man to wear a girdle may sound utterly ridiculous . . . but once most men with angina try it for a week, they realize that they are less fatigued and suffer fewer angina attacks, says Dr. Steincrohn. Wearing a girdle that provides support of the "pot belly" seems to be an easy and inexpensive way to reduce angina.

• For some angina patients, an aspirin a day can reduce the chance of having a heart attack, the Food and Drug Administration (FDA) says. One aspirin tablet per day can cut heart attacks by 20% for some people who have already had heart attacks to as much as 50% in men who have unstable angina. In patients with unstable angina, an aspirin a day reduced the risk of getting a heart attack or of dying of a heart attack by about half, according to the FDA. During the three-month study in those with unstable angina, the risk of having a heart attack was lowered from a 12% chance without aspirin, to a 6% chance with aspirin. Aspirin is not a substitute for other preventative therapies for heart attacks, cautions FDA commissioner Frank E. Young, M.D. He advises that patients consult their physicians before starting daily aspirin for angina.

• Vitamin E may play a role in helping to reduce angina pain. At the University of British Columbia in Canada, Dr. Terence W. Anderson has done preliminary tests involving angina patients and vitamin E supplements. Although it was a small study including just 15 patients, Dr. Anderson found that angina pain increased when vitamin E supplements were switched to a placebo. The patients did not know their medication was changed. However, every man whose vitamin E was switched asked to be taken out of the study because of an increase in angina pain. Whole-grain products, green vegetables, milk, almonds, peanuts, pecans, soybeans, eggs and meat are good natural sources of vitamin E, but taking large doses of vitamin E can be dangerous.

• People receiving digitalis or other heart medication should not take calcium ascorbate (a vitamin C formulation), since irregular heartbeats may occur.

Here are some general recommendations to improve your overall health and to help reduce your angina symptoms:

> Lose weight. Be kind to your heart.

> Don't eat too much at one sitting. Overeating or eating at irregular times can disrupt your body and put extra stress on the heart. Take a rest for at least half an hour after eating.

> Stop smoking. Smoking causes a buildup of plaque in your heart arteries.

> Exercise. Gradually increasing the amount of light, aerobic exercise, like walking, that you get will help strengthen your heart and arteries. Check with your doctor for an exercise schedule.

> Get proper rest and a good night's sleep. To get a good supply of oxygen and fresh air for the night's rest, open the windows wide for about 10 minutes, then leave them open about an inch. A stuffy room may inhibit your ability to sleep, according to Dr. Charles Wolfe, Jr. of the Sleep Disorder Center in Chicago.

Arthritis

Learning to live with arthritis can be difficult. There is no known cure for arthritis. However, many of the discomforts of arthritis can be reduced by taking special care of yourself.

• Maintain your ideal weight. Obesity places additional strain on inflamed joints. A weight reduction diet may be recommended by your doctor to reduce excess pressure on the joints.

• Exercise your muscles and joints every day. Simple exercises, like rotating the feet and stretching the muscles, should be done for short periods of time and repeated throughout the day. Long sets of strenuous exercise or contact sports can harm the joints. Good general exercises are walking, hiking, swimming, bicycling and low-impact aerobics. Many local pools offer "exercising in water" classes for arthritis sufferers. Always warm-up before starting vigorous activities by doing some slow stretching exercises. Be sure to end an exercise session with the same type of cooling down, slow stretches.

• Use heat or cold treatments to help reduce pain and swelling. Some people find heat works best for them, whereas other people experience the most relief from cold. Many prefer alternating between hot and cold treatments. Hot-water bottles, heating pads, paraffin wax treatments, hot compresses, 250-watt reflector heat lamps, bath and showers are excellent sources of heat. Moist heat is usually preferred rather than dry heat. Don't use the heat for more than twenty minutes at a sitting, because after that time the heat loses its effectiveness. Never use a hair dryer, sun lamp, tanning booth, or ultraviolet light to provide heat.

• Learn to rest. Don't push yourself. Take breaks from long activities. A proper balance between exercise and rest is best for the joints. Many people find that their pain improves significantly when they increase the number of hours they sleep each night.

• Learn to manage the stress in your life. Stress can contribute to joint pain because the muscles become tense with stress. Tense muscles have a more difficult time supporting the joints, and the joints will become tender. Stress can also reduce your overall health which will negatively affect your arthritis symptoms.

• Set reasonable goals for yourself. The time it takes you to complete a project may be a lot longer now than before you had arthritis. Don't place yourself under additional stress by setting unrealistic goals.

• Plan the priorities in your life and work to achieve those. Learn to "conserve your energy" for things that are important to you. Planning events while remembering your needs as an arthritic, can help make the most of special and everyday events.

• Develop a positive attitude. Learn to focus on the things you <u>can</u> do rather than dwelling on the pain and limitations arthritis brings. By remaining socially active and concentrating on other things, you can learn to live with your arthritis. Find ways you can help others. This will not only benefit them but will contribute to your own sense of worth and value.

• Respect your pain. Many times people ignore their pain and continue doing harmful activities. You should learn to use your pain to tell you when to slow down. Learn when to quit what you are doing and rest before overexertion and unnecessary soreness set in.

• Consider a fat-free diet. Researchers at Wayne State University Medical School in Michigan tested a small group of people with rheumatoid arthritis on a fat-free diet. Within seven weeks, <u>all</u> of the arthritis had gone into remission. This was only a small test, but a fat-free diet may be worth a try. A fat-free diet may help your arthritis, your heart, your arteries and could help you lose weight.

• Sometimes allergy to a specific food causes arthritic-like symptoms. If you suspect that a certain food is causing your problems, try keeping food and arthritis charts for about two months. On one chart keep track of everything you eat and drink each day. On the other chart, record all of your arthritis symptoms, when they occurred, what joints were affected, and how long they lasted. At the end of two months, see if you can notice any correlations between the two charts. Then try and eliminate any suspect foods from your diet. Continue working on both diaries and note any changes in your arthritis.

• Weather or climate have NOT been proven to affect arthritis. If you feel that a warmer or drier climate is more suitable for you, consider a long visit before you make a permanent move. However, there is no medical evidence that the climate cures or improves arthritis.

• Use your joints carefully to prevent them from further damage. Always use the largest possible joint or number of joints for each task. For example, use your whole hand, instead of just your fingers. Carry things carefully. Supporting something with two hands may reduce the strain of carrying an object.

• Strive to obtain good posture while sitting or standing. Good posture will improve the muscles' ability to support the joints and will help prevent deformities from occurring.

• Take advantage of the many new products for arthritis sufferers. Wide handles, easy-to-open containers, velcro fasteners, elastic shoelaces, buttoning aids and many other inventions can make your life easier.

• Sleep on a firm, comfortable mattress. Some people like a firm water bed that can be heated. One company has just designed a special mattress, made from weaving wool, that has been tested by arthritics and people with back problems. Ninety percent of the people in the mattress test found that the new mattress improved their sleep and reduced their arthritis symptoms. Woolrest® is the brand name of this weaving wool mattress.

• Don't sleep on your stomach. This position can damage the alignment of your neck and back.

• If you suffer from stiff hands in the morning, try wearing gloves to bed. Dr. Frank Schmid, in a study for the Arthritis Foundation, discovered that wearing stretch gloves decreased the amount of swelling, numbness and stiffness in arthritic hands.

• Try sleeping in a sleeping bag, with an electric blanket or on a heated water bed to reduce morning stiffness.

• Enjoy a warm bath or shower as soon as you get out of bed. Do gentle stretching exercises while in the water, or just after you finish. While the muscles are warm from the water, they are easier to stretch.

• For severe morning stiffness, you may want to set your alarm clock half an hour early. If you take an aspirin about 30 minutes before you want to get out of bed, the aspirin will have time to reduce the swelling and pain. Be sure to sit up when swallowing the aspirin or other arthritis medication. (Never take a pill while lying down as it could get caught in the throat.)

• In some severe cases, people have experienced relief from arthritis by being hypnotized. Hypnosis can help the person relax and temporarily cope with the pain.

• Do not stay in the same position for extended periods of time. Holding a telephone during a long conversation can cause your fingers to become swollen and stiff. If you are sitting for a long time, get up and walk around every hour of so. Do needlework and other intense projects in short spurts so you don't stay in the same position for hours on end.

• Beware of "false" arthritis. Self-diagnosis can be harmful. If you suspect that you have arthritis (see symptoms following), be sure to see your doctor. Sometimes people who are experiencing joint pain, inflammation or swelling are really suffering from the side effects of their prescription drugs. Several common drugs can cause arthritis-like symptoms including Tagamet® (cimetidine), beta blockers like Lopressor® (metoprolol), iron supplements, barbiturates, blood-pressure reducers, sulfa drugs, quinidine, penicillamine, diuretics, amphotericin B and tetracycline.

• Other drugs may aggravate systemic lupus erythematosus, a form of arthritis commonly known as lupus. Oral contraceptives, Apresoline®, penicillin, tetracycline, some sulfa drugs and several anti-cancer drugs can increase the symptoms of lupus.

• If there is a history of arthritis in your family, you should be aware of the early warning signs of arthritis as described by the Arthritis Foundation. If you notice any of these symptoms, discuss them with your doctor.

> Nagging pain and stiffness in the morning
> Redness or warmth in a joint
> Pain or tenderness in one or more joints
> Not being able to move a joint normally
> Swelling in one or more joints
> Pain and stiffness in the neck, lower back, knees or other joints
> Tingling sensations in the fingertips, hands or feet
> Unexplained weight loss, fever, weakness or tiredness

• Your doctor will want to know several things before he or she can work out an arthritis-care program for you.

> How long are the flare-ups?
> What joints are affected?

> Is it worse in the morning or later in the day?

> Is there any redness or swelling at the site of the soreness?

> Is there any fever or temperature increase overall?

Also see: **Gout.**

Asthma

Be sure to read the section on **Airborne Allergies.** Many of the preventative measures for airborne allergies also apply to people with asthma.

• Asthmatics should practice methods to relieve stress. Asthma is not a psychological disorder. However, strong emotions like stress, worry and fear can trigger an asthma attack. The emotions don't cause the disease itself, but they can aggravate it. Deep breathing exercises and relaxation techniques may help reduce the severity of an attack.

• Yoga exercises may help. According to a study published in the British Medical Journal (1/19/85), asthmatics who practiced yoga exercises for at least six months suffered fewer asthma attacks. The researchers believe that yoga helps to relax the nervous system, which lowers the intensity and frequency of asthma attacks.

• Vigorous exercise, such as running, or drastic changes in temperature can trigger an attack. An estimated 85% of asthmatics have symptoms of wheezing after exercise, according to the American Academy of Allergy and Immunology. Exercise that requires hard breathing for long periods of time (like long-distance running) and most activities in cold air should be avoided. Swimming is good exercise for an asthmatic because it provides overall body exercise, yet the asthmatic's air passages will not dry out due to lack of moisture.

• Do not eat ice cream or drink extremely cold liquids because your bronchial tubes may be shocked into spasms by the cold.

• Avoid foods containing yellow dye #5. Between 47,000 and 94,000 asthmatics in the U.S. are affected by this food coloring known as tartrazine yellow. Many other food additives, like BHA and BHT, may aggravate asthma. To avoid dyes and additives, try to eat non-processed, natural foods when possible. Wash all fruit and vegetables thoroughly before eating. Unfortunately, this will not remove all the chemicals used during growing and transporting, but washing can remove some of them.

• Asthmatics need to avoid beta-blocking drugs or use them only with extreme caution. Beta-blockers, used to help treat high blood pressure, can constrict the bronchial muscles and cause life-threatening problems for an asthmatic. Beta-blockers are widely prescribed and include:

acebutolol (Sectral®), atenolol (Tenormin®), metoprolol (Lopressor®), nadolol (Corgard®), pindolol (Visken®), propranolol (Inderal®), and timolol (Blocadren®). Be sure you and your doctor have thoroughly considered both your asthma and your blood pressure problems. Do not stop taking any medication without your physician's approval.

• Timolol (Timoptic®) eye drops, used to treat glaucoma and pressure in the eye, have been associated with at least five deaths of asthmatics. Timoptic® is applied directly to the eye and is available only by prescription. Notify your eye doctor if you have asthma and are taking this medication.

• Penicillin, aspirin and many other anti- inflammatory drugs can cause severe asthma attacks. Some of these drugs are known as NSAIDs (Non-Steroidal Anti-Inflammatory Drugs). NSAIDs are commonly used to help treat arthritis, menstrual cramps and general pain. Ibuprofen is a NSAID that is available without prescription as Advil®, Haltran®, Medipren®, Nuprin®, Trendar® and several other brands. It is also available in stronger doses, by prescription only, as Motrin® and Rufen®. Other NSAIDs, available only with a prescription, are: ketoprofen (Orudis®), indomethacin (Indocin®), naproxen (Naprosyn®), mefenamic acid (Ponstel®), sulindac (Clinoril®), piroxicam (Feldene®), and suprofen (Suprol®).

• Ozone, sulfur dioxide, nitrogen dioxide, cigarette smoke, carbon monoxide, hydrocarbons, nitrogen oxide and photochemical substances are air pollutants that can trigger asthma attacks. Follow the air pollution index reports in your area and stay indoors when the levels are high.

Back Problems

• Avoid moving suddenly. Sharp or sudden movements can aggravate back pain. Getting out of a car too quickly after sitting still for a long time or jumping up to answer the phone can be very dangerous for back problems. Learn to move slowly and carefully.

• Straining your neck muscles can aggravate your back. Don't hold the phone between your neck and your ear, even with a phone rest. Always hold the phone with your hand to avoid tensing up the neck muscles.

• Be careful when doing housework. We often underestimate how difficult housework is. Be sure to take breaks between doing heavy tasks. Stretch your back and neck muscles, as you would before exercising. By stretching them before the heavy tasks you will help prepare them and could avoid unnecessary muscle strain.

• Push, don't pull. Pulling heavy objects creates

more strain on your lower back than pushing the object. If you suffer from back problems, don't be afraid to ask for help to move large objects.

• Move around frequently. Don't stay in one position for a long period of time. If you are driving, flying in an airplane or working at a desk, be sure to get up at least once each hour. Take a walk or change positions often.

• Always read in a comfortable position. Rest your arms on your lap, the arms of your chair, a table or a desk while reading.

• Take breaks from any repetitious activity. A housewife suffered severe neck and back pain from doing needlework. Each night while cross-stitching, she held her head slightly to the side and did not support her arms. She remained in the same position for at least five hours each day. Now, after spending several weeks in a neck brace to reduce the pain, she cross-stitches only for short periods of time.

• Watch your posture. Don't slouch or sit in extremely soft chairs or couches. Be sure your back is properly supported whenever you are sitting or lying down. When driving or riding in a car, tilt the seat slightly forward. At first this position may feel awkward, but it will give you better support and posture while in the car.

• Exercise. Regular exercise will help strengthen

the back muscles so they will not be strained or aggravated by regular activities. When exercising, try to avoid sudden, jarring movements. Always warm up before starting vigorous exercise and use slow stretching exercises to cool-down afterwards. If using aerobic dance for exercise, try low-impact aerobics which keep one foot on the floor at all times, causing less jumping and jarring of the joints. A proper low-impact program will still give a good aerobic work-out while lowering the possibility of damaging your back.

• Strengthen your lower back muscles by holding in your stomach and buttock muscles to a count of ten. Release and tighten again. Repeat this several times each day to help strengthen the back muscles.

• To relieve lower back pain, soak in a warm bathtub or apply a heating pad directly to the back. Lie down on a firm surface and relax while applying gentle heat to the area. Try to avoid lying directly on a heating pad. It is best to put the heating pad on top of the body. If you must lie with it underneath, keep the heating pad on the lowest setting and use it for no more than 20 minutes.

Blood Pressure — High
• Most people diagnosed as having high blood

pressure are instructed to go on a low salt (low sodium) diet, but sodium is found in many other items than just table salt. People on low-sodium diets should also avoid taking sodium ascorbate. Sodium ascorbate is a formulation of vitamin C that contains sodium. If you need a vitamin C supplement while cutting back on sodium, ascorbic acid or calcium ascorbate forms of vitamin C are preferred.

If you still crave spicy food but are trying to reduce salt, try putting lemon juice on your food instead. Several salt-free mixtures of herbs and spices are also available for seasonings. Most people find that once they eliminate salt and get over the initial craving for salt, they don't miss it. The preference for salt is something our taste buds learned as we grew up with highly salted foods.

• Avoid all forms of tobacco. Smoking is a well-known hazard to people with high blood pressure. Smoking cigarettes, pipes or cigars can clog the arteries, which raises blood pressure and increases the risk of heart failure. Chewing tobacco, plugs and snuff, known as smokeless tobacco, should also be avoided because of their high salt content. According to an article in the New England Journal of Medicine (312 : 919) the sodium levels in chewing tobacco and snuff are similar to the high levels found in dill pickles. Studies at Ohio State

University have shown higher blood pressure levels in people who used smokeless tobacco, compared to nonusers. Smokeless tobacco also contains high amounts of licorice. Licorice should be avoided because it causes the body to hold onto sodium, lose potassium and retain fluids.

• One research study shows that listening, rather than talking, lowers blood pressure. Most people experience a rise in blood pressure when they speak, followed by a rapid drop when they listen, reports Arteries Cleaned Out Naturally. The study indicates that the louder and faster a person talks, the higher the blood pressure. Learning to listen may reduce stress and the load on the heart.

• Inderal® and other beta-blocking drugs, prescribed to help lower high blood pressure, may cause depression, according to a study in the Journal of the American Medical Association (JAMA 255: 357-360). More than 20 percent of people taking beta-blockers eventually start taking antidepressant drugs, says Dr. Jerry Avorn of Harvard Medical School, who conducted the study. Dr. Avorn says this is the first study that linked depression and beta-blockers although many doctors have suspected a connection for several years. If you suspect your medication is causing your depression, discuss it with your doctor. Never stop taking a prescribed drug without your doctor's consent.

• People with high blood pressure should avoid overeating when they are on antidepressant drugs. Unusual feelings of hunger and cravings for sweets are experienced by about 50% of people taking drugs for depression, according to the journal Geriatrics (41:4). The unusual cravings often cause people to eat more than normal and to gain weight. Being overweight is dangerous for everyone, but especially for those with high blood pressure. The pangs of hunger and cravings for sweets seem to be side effects of antidepressant drugs that stop as soon as the drug is discontinued, says the report. If you suspect that your prescription drugs are causing these side effects, discuss them with your doctor. Do NOT stop or change your medicine without your physician's approval.

• Here are some tips for people taking medicine to control high blood pressure:

> Get your blood pressure checked regularly; it takes only a minute or two. If it is above the normal range (140/90), see your doctor.

> Take your prescribed medicine as directed. Keep doing so, because even if you feel better, your high blood pressure is not cured. Regular dosages are necessary to keep it under control.

> Don't change the dose yourself. You might get too much or not enough medicine. Either way it

could be harmful. If you take less of your prescription than your doctor prescribes, you may increase the risk of complications such as stroke or heart attack. If you take more of your medication than you're supposed to, you increase the possibility of having side effects from the drug.

> Don't stop taking a drug on your own, even if you feel lightheaded, dizzy, tired, depressed or have trouble sleeping. Your drug can be controlling your blood pressure but may also be giving you these or other side effects. Notify your doctor immediately when bothersome side effects occur. He needs to know how medication is affecting you, in order to treat your condition properly.

> If you have questions about your high blood pressure or your prescription, don't ask a friend or relative. Their information or advice may be well-intended but wrong for you. Ask your doctor or pharmacist — they are the people qualified to answer.

> Be sure to tell your doctor if you take other medicine regularly. Prescription drugs, vitamins, aspirin and other non-prescription drugs can interact with one another, causing decreased effectiveness or problem side effects.

> Proper diet and exercise often help control high blood pressure. Consult your doctor to see how you can help lower your high blood

pressure... maybe to the point where drugs aren't needed!

• If you suffer, or have suffered, from high blood pressure, be careful with your children's intake of salt, according to research published in the journal <u>Pediatrics</u> (June 1980). Craving salt is an acquired taste. Do not salt your children's food. Limit the amount of salt you use in food preparation. Limit the children's intake of highly salted foods like canned soups, potato chips, pickles and cured meats. If children do not grow up with salt, they will not crave it, and you will lower their risk of getting high blood pressure in the future.

Blood Pressure — Low

Before you shower after exercising, cool down, warns Dr. John Cantwell in the <u>American Medical Journal</u> (252:429). Cantwell, the team doctor for the Atlanta Braves baseball club, says that showering too soon after exercising can cause a sharp decrease in blood pressure. Exercise itself causes a fall in blood pressure because, after exercise, the blood tends to collect in the legs, he explains. If you take a hot or warm shower while in this condition, the hot water can dilate the blood vessels and create an even greater drop in blood pressure. On the other hand, a cold shower can raise blood pressure too quickly, placing a sudden strain on the heart that could cause some arteries to go into spasms, explains the doctor. To avoid any bad effects, Dr. Cantwell recommends that after exercising, you should completely cool down before heading for the shower.

Body Odor

Proper hygiene is the best prevention against strong body odor. However, some people tend to give off an offensive odor even if their personal hygiene habits are excellent.

Avoid washing and bathing too much. Daily showers or baths may dry out the skin and reduce the body's natural oils. The natural oils help to control body odor because without them the body's natural defenses are lowered, and the odor increases. A complete bath twice a week is adequate for many people unless your skin is very oily. Washing the face, feet, armpits, rectum and genitals should be done daily.

Breath — Shortness of

• Shortness of breath due to stress or anxiety can be a very frightening experience. As we start to hyperventilate or "overbreathe", the level of carbon dioxide in the blood drops, and dizziness, lightheadedness, nausea and tingling sensations can set in. Trying to take slow, deep breaths may help at a time like this. Try inhaling as you silently count to 10, hold it for 5 seconds, then breathe out to another count of 10. At first, the breaths may be much shorter. However, if you concentrate and try to relax, deep breathing can restore the carbon dioxide level and relieve the problems.

Bruce Hensel, M.D., a professor at UCLA, suggests breathing into a paper bag for several minutes. The paper bag treatment will also raise the carbon dioxide level. This is especially good for people who cannot achieve slow, deep breathing on their own.

• If you wake up during the night because of shortness of breath, see your doctor as soon as possible. Sudden shortness of breath could be caused by asthma, a lung problem or heart trouble.

Bronchitis   See: Lung Diseases

Bruises

Easy bruising may be caused by a deficiency of vitamins K or C. Vitamin K is naturally found in green, leafy vegetables, fruits, cereals, dairy products and meats. Vitamin C is obtained from citrus fruit, rose hips, acerola cherries, green peppers, parsley, broccoli, Brussels sprouts, cabbage and potatoes.

Being bruised easily may also be a sign of a more serious health problem. You should see your doctor for her opinion.

Burn Treatment

• Serious burns should be treated by a physician. Minor burns may be treated at home only if the epidermis, the outer layer of the skin, is burned without blistering. Minor burns are classified as first degree burns; second and third degree burns are more serious. Minor burns are usually caused by touching a hot object, hot water or steam, or getting a sunburn.

According to The American Medical Association's Handbook of First Aid and Emergency Care, minor burns should be placed under cold running water immediately or covered by a cold compress to relieve the pain. Next, the burn should be covered with clean bandages to protect it from infection.

The American Medical Association (AMA) does not recommend putting butter, grease, lard, ointments or any other substance on a burn without your doctor's recommendation.

• For burns caused by a chemical, it is important to hold the burned area under cool running water for at least five minutes. This is also true if your eye has been burned by a chemical. Flushing the burned area or the eye with water will help dilute the chemical and prevent the burn from getting any worse. Do this first before calling a doctor or have someone else call for help, so the area can be cleansed as soon as possible.

• Additional vitamin C may help healing after a burn Dr. James Wasco reports in Woman's Day magazine. Dr. Wasco recommends taking 500 mg. of vitamin C twice daily to help heal burns, fractures or other damage to the body tissues.

Cancer

• The American Cancer Society has developed a list of seven warning signs of cancer. Using the letters of the word CAUTION, they are easy to remember. If you notice any of these signs in yourself or a loved one, contact your doctor immediately. Early detection of cancer saves lives.

C —Change in the color or size of a wart or mole.

A —A sore that will not heal or is slow to heal.

U —Unusual, irregular or unexplained bleeding

in the bowels, urine, nipples or vagina.

T —Thickening or lump in the breast, lip, tongue or elsewhere.

I —Indigestion or difficulty swallowing.

O —Obvious change in bowel or bladder habits.

N —Nagging or persistent cough or hoarseness.

• Common skin tags may be a warning signal of colon cancer. Skin tags are small lesions, usually occurring in groups in the neck, armpits and groin areas. Until now, skin tags were thought to be harmless but cosmetically annoying. Researchers at the Mount Sinai School of Medicine in New York have discovered that 86 percent of their patients with colon cancer polyps also had skin tags. In further testing, 69 percent of their patients with skin tags, also had colon polyps. The researchers at Mount Sinai suggest that, to be safe, anyone with skin tags should have their stools checked for blood. You may want to ask your pharmacist about over-the-counter stool tests that can be done in the privacy of your own home. Since a stool test is a simple and inexpensive procedure, it would be best to be safe and have the test either at home or at your doctor's office.

• Cancer tumors in the mouth can be reduced or prevented by beta-carotene, based on the results of preliminary research at Harvard University. Beta-carotene is a natural substance found in fruits and vegetables, especially in yellow vegetables like carrots. The healthy human body produces vitamin A from beta-carotene. According to the Harvard study, published in the journal <u>Carcinogenesis</u>, cancer tumors in hamsters' mouths disappeared within two weeks after a beta-carotene solution had been applied directly onto the tumors or injected into the tumors. Other research, including more work at Harvard, has shown that people who eat fruits and vegetables high in carotene seem to have a lower than normal incidence of cancer.

• Ultraviolet rays from sunshine are being blamed again for causing cancer. We know that we should protect our skin and eyes from exposure to ultraviolet rays. Now, new research at Cornell University suggests that ultraviolet rays actually destroy beta-carotene. As mentioned, beta-carotene is used by the body to create vitamin A, which has natural anti-cancer properties to help prevent lung cancer, bladder cancer and skin cancer.

Please protect yourself against cancer: use a sunscreen with a SPF (sun protection factor) of at least 12, protect your eyes with high quality sunglasses, and avoid unnecessary exposure to ultraviolet light.

• Vitamin C may play a role in the treatment or prevention of cancer. Terminal cancer patients, with cancer so advanced that other treatments had been abandoned, were given vitamin C. In studies by Linus Pauling, the patients who received the vitamin supplementation lived a few more months before dying (a dubious benefit) than those not given vitamin C. If you have cancer, do not stop or change the treatment prescribed by your doctor, but you may want to discuss the benefits of vitamin C supplementation.

Vitamin C is an antioxidant that may slow down certain cell chemistry functions, such as increased harmful peroxidation and free-radical formation. It is thought that free-radicals play a major role in causing cancer, heart disease, hardening of the arteries and aging.

Vitamin C may offer protection from some cancer-causing substances. Nitrates and nitrites, commonly used in food preservation, combine with amino acids in the body to form nitrosamines. Nitrosamines are thought to be cancer-causing substances. Vitamin C, according to <u>Vitamin Side Effects Revealed</u>, is thought to prevent this combination from taking place. The National Academy of Science Committee on Diet, Nutrition and Cancer states: "Vitamin C can inhibit the formation of some carcinogens (cancer-causing substances) . . . The consumption of vitamin C containing foods is associated with a lower risk of cancers of the stomach and esophagus." In separate research, women with low levels of vitamin C were shown to have an increased incidence of precancerous abnormalities of the cervix. Doctors are not necessarily recommending increased supplementation of vitamin C, but they do recommend eating more foods that are rich in vitamin C such as: rose hips, acerola cherries, citrus fruits, green peppers, parsley, broccoli, Brussels sprouts, cabbage, and potatoes. Cooking causes 50-55% of the vitamin to be lost, so raw fruit and vegetables are best. Fresh, refrigerated or frozen juices have higher amounts of vitamin C than canned juices.

• Your fiber intake should be at least 30 grams each day, according to the National Cancer Institute. For the best overall effect, your diet should include a variety of fruits, miller's bran, oat bran, vegetables, whole-grain breads and cereals .

• Exercise may lower your risk of getting certain cancers, according to the New England Journal of Medicine (314, 10: 605). Women who participated in college sports and continue to exercise regularly have a lower incidence of uterine, vaginal, cervical, ovarian and breast cancer than women who are not exercising. This study by Harvard University's Grace Wyshak, Ph.D. and Rose Frisch, Ph.D. involved over 5,000 women.

• High amounts of fat in your diet, if you are a woman, could double your chances of getting ovarian cancer, according to research from the Boston Hospital for Women. Women who drank skim milk, ate fish, used margarine and used vegetable oil to replace animal fat had a lower than average incidence of ovarian cancer. Drinking whole milk and eating animal fat and butter all increase the amount of fat in your diet. Reducing the amount of fat in the diet may help lower the risk of ovarian cancer, says another study which was published in <u>Obstetrics and Gynecology</u> (63:833). This study supports the findings of Dr. David A. Snowden from the University of Minnesota. In Dr. Snowden's study, women who ate eggs or fried foods died from ovarian cancer at three times the ovarian cancer death rate of women who avoided eggs and fried foods.

• Women with a history of breast cancer in their familes should be especially careful to give themselves monthly breast exams and have regular breast exams and mammograms by their physicians. According to statistics from the Centers for Disease Control in Atlanta (<u>Journal of the American Medical Association</u> JAMA 253 :1908), women who have a mother **and** a sister with breast cancer have 14 times the normal risk of developing breast cancer. If a grandmother or aunt has had breast cancer, their risk is 1.5 times greater than average. If a mother **or** a sister has had it, the risk is 2.3 times greater. Women with a family history of breast cancer should alert their doctors. Careful screening and early detection should help keep an occurrence of breast cancer as limited as possible.

In a monthly self-exam, a woman's breasts need to be checked for all warning signs of cancer, not just lumps. Dr. James Wasco, M.D., a columnist for Woman's Day magazine, reports that several other things can be possible warning signals. As you begin regular monthly breast exams, you will be able to catch any changes much earlier than your doctor. You will be familiar with the shape, normal lumps and coloring of your own breasts. During your monthly self-exam watch for:

> Any change in the shape, size or color of the breasts. Do this by comparing them in a mirror each month. Compare them to each other and to how they looked in the previous month.

> Any unusual discharge should be noted and reported to your doctor.

> Scaliness or crustiness on the breasts, especially around the nipple.

> Any new dimples in the breasts.

> Any lumps or thickening of the breast tissue.

> Asymmetry — any difference in the shapes of the breasts.

Canker Sores

A canker sore is a tiny, raw ulcer located on the tissue inside the mouth. They are usually quite painful and can occur inside the cheeks or lips, on the gums and under the tongue.

• Some doctors believe that canker sores are caused by a deficiency of vitamin B12 (cobalamin), iron and folic acid. Vitamin B12 is found naturally in liver, meat, milk, dairy products, fish and eggs. It is virtually absent in vegetables. Many vegetarians who do not eat meat or eggs may have a vitamin B12 deficiency. Folic acid is found in yeast, liver, lima beans, whole-grain products, leafy green vegetables, asparagus, beans, turnips, peanuts, oats, potatoes and oranges. Folic acid and vitamin B12 work together. If there is a low amount of one of these vitamins in the diet, the other one will not work as well. Iron is found in whole-grain products, liver, organ meats, red meat, eggs, lima beans, prunes, spinach, raw broccoli, peas, fish and raisins.

• A diet high in lysine and low in arginine may help reduce canker sores. Studies at Indiana University School of Medicine and at UCLA have found that lysine helps repress the sores and arginine promotes their growth. Both lysine and arginine are amino acids. Dairy products and yeast are high in lysine. Nuts, seeds, chocolate and some cereals are high in arginine and low in lysine and should be avoided, according to the research. Some doctors recommend lysine supplements up to 1,200 milligrams daily to help stop canker sores.

Cholesterol Reduction

Reducing blood cholesterol levels will help reduce the rate of coronary heart disease and hardening of the arteries. Researchers have observed that the levels of fats in the blood can be lowered by changes in the diet. As early as 1947, a study of seven nations showed a direct relationship between a country's incidence of heart disease, the level of cholesterol in the blood and the amount of animal fat in the national diet.

Only extremely high cholesterol levels require drug therapy. Clinical tests indicate that each one-percent reduction in blood cholesterol levels nets a two-percent reduction in coronary heart disease rates. For example, a five-percent reduction in blood-cholesterol levels should reduce coronary heart disease rates by ten-percent.

The first step in lowering blood cholesterol levels is diet therapy and weight loss, if you are overweight. A moderate exercise program may also be helpful. The dietary approach is to lower total fat, saturated fat and cholesterol consumption. Here are some suggestions:

> Saturated fats, found in meats and dairy products, should be reduced to less than 10% of total calories. Foods that are rich in cholesterol, and should be avoided or drastically limited in the diet, are: egg yolks, organ meats and most cheeses. Foods that should be reduced because they are high in saturated fats include: butter, bacon, beef, whole milk, cream, chocolate, almost any food of animal origin, hydrogenated vegetable shortenings, coconut oil and palm oil.

> Unsaturated fats, such as fish and vegetable oils, may constitute only as much as 10% of total calories.

> Total fat intake should be less than 30% of your daily calories.

> Do not consume more than 100 milligrams of cholesterol for each 1,000 calories. Daily cholesterol should not exceed 300 milligrams.

> Cut back on beef, lamb and pork. Never eat any combination of them more than three times per week.

If you must eat beef, stick to lean cuts. At home, cut off all visible fat. Broiling, baking or roasting meat in its own juice are the most healthful methods of preparation. When eating out, lean cuts like filet mignon or chateaubriand are best. Keep your portions small and don't use gravy or cream sauce.

Also avoid casseroles and pot pies.

> Don't eat duck or goose. Both are high in fat content.

> Replace red meat with turkey, veal, fish, seafood and chicken. Be sure to cut off the skin before you prepare chicken or turkey because much of the fat is contained in the skin. Eat the light meat on poultry since it contains less fat than the dark meat.

> Avoid prepared luncheon meats. They are high in fat, sodium and nitrites. Sliced turkey breast, tuna salad and salmon salad (without mayonnaise) are good luncheon alternatives.

> Limit your egg yolks to two per week. This includes not only whole eggs, but eggs used in baking and cooking. The American Heart Association recommends making this cholesterol-free egg substitute, especially for use in baking: Beat three egg whites. Then add 1/4 cup non-fat milk, 1 tablespoon non-fat dry milk powder, and 1 teaspoon of polyunsaturated vegetable oil. Mix these four ingredients together to make a healthful egg substitute. According to an avid cholesterol-watcher, if you add a drop of yellow food coloring to this mixture when making French toast, your family won't be able to tell the difference!

> If you buy a ready-made egg substitute, make sure that it is cholesterol-free and fat-free.

> Pre-packaged cake mixes, biscuits and pancake

mixes are usually made with eggs in their mixtures. To make your own easy mix, combine all the necessary dry ingredients together and freeze. When you want to bake them, just take your mix out of the freezer and add the liquids. For the liquids, use only egg substitutes, non-fat milk or vegetable oils.

> When buying pasta, avoid noodles made with eggs.

> Avoid crackers that contain lard. Study the list of ingredients and buy only crackers made with acceptable vegetable oils. If a warm cracker leaves a grease stain on a paper towel, it contains too much fat.

> Avoid croissants.

> When buying bagels, choose those made with water rather than with eggs.

> Switch from butter to margarine.

> For sautéing, use a vegetable spray. The spray will limit the amount of fat you'll use in cooking.

> Avoid butter or sour cream on baked potatoes. A plain, low-fat baked potato is good for you.

> Substitute low-fat cottage cheese or nonfat, plain yogurt for sour cream in your favorite recipes.

> Use a salt substitute or herbs on your popcorn instead of salt and butter.

> If you want cheese, eat just a little of the low-fat varieties like Mozzarella, Provolone and Swiss.

For the taste of cheese, try a sprinkle of grated Parmesan cheese. It will still give you a cheese flavor, but it contains fewer grams of fat.

> Avoid heavy salad dressings like blue cheese. Try to eat less salad dressing by placing the dressing on the side and using it as a "dip".

> Drink skim or low-fat milk. Avoid using whole milk, evaporated milk or sweetened condensed milk.

> Do not use artificial creamers because they are high in unwanted fats. For convenience, use an evaporated low-fat milk powder in your coffee.

> Switch from ice cream to sorbet or frozen fruit treats. Beware of frozen yogurt unless it is frozen low-fat yogurt.

> Limit your intake of chocolate. Substitute cocoa powder for chocolate (when possible) in recipes. The American Heart Association suggests substituting three tablespoons cocoa powder and one tablespoon polyunsaturated oil for each one ounce piece of baking chocolate to cut the amount of saturated fat by over 60%.

> Vegetable oils that are recommended for a low-fat diet include corn, safflower, cottonseed, sunflower, soybean and sesame seed oil.

• One of the best sources of beneficial "omega 3" polyunsaturated fats is fish, especially cold water fish like salmon, trout, mackerel and cod.

Researchers are discovering that fish oils actually lower levels of cholesterol and other blood fats associated with heart disease. New fish oil supplements are available on the market, but they may contain too much vitamin A, which can be toxic or too little of the beneficial omega 3 fatty acids. Until studies have proven their safety and effectiveness, it is probably better to eat fish than take fish oil supplements.

• Walnuts and pecans are high in polyunsaturates. Chestnuts are also a healthful snack because they are low in fat.

• The way food is prepared can make a big difference in the amount of fat it contains. At home or in a restaurant, try to eat foods in their most natural form. Foods that are broiled, steamed, roasted or baked in their own juices will contain less fat than foods that are cooked in other ways.

• Avoid foods that are fried, sautéed, breaded, "buttery", or "crispy".

• Avoid all foods prepared with sauce or gravy like cheese sauce (described as "au gratin"), hollandaise sauce, lobster sauce, sweet and sour sauce, mayonnaise or regular gravy.

• A diet well-balanced in fiber is thought to help reduce cholesterol levels. Pectin, a type of fiber found in fruits and oat bran, is an excellent source of fiber that may reduce cholesterol levels. In studies at Northwestern University and the Lipid Research Clinic, eating oat bran lowered cholesterol levels dramatically in just a few weeks. Fruit, miller's bran, vegetables, oat bran, brown rice, whole-grain breads and cereals are good sources of dietary fiber.

• Eating certain foods can help lower your cholesterol levels, according to Dr. Frank Field in <u>Family Circle</u> magazine. Dr. Field suggests that many people know what foods to reduce in their diet, but most people do not know what foods they should increase in their diets. To lower your cholesterol level, he recommends increasing your intake of:

> apples and oranges
> all fruits and vegetables (fresh or frozen varieties are best)
> olive oil and corn oil
> kidney beans especially, and all dried beans, including pinto beans, garbanzo beans, chickpeas, navy beans and lentils
> oat bran
> whole grains, cereal, brown rice and egg-free pasta.
> salmon.

• Vitamin C is an antioxidant that may slow down certain cell chemistry functions, such as increased harmful peroxidation and free-radical formation.

It is thought that free-radicals play a major role in causing hardening of the arteries, heart disease, cancer and aging. Vitamin C is naturally obtained from citrus fruit, berries, rose hips, acerola cherries, green peppers, parsley, broccoli, brussels sprouts, cabbage and potatoes.

• Niacin (vitamin B3) given in high doses has been shown to reduce the amount of cholesterol in the blood (<u>Journal</u> <u>of</u> <u>the</u> <u>American</u> <u>Medical</u> <u>Association</u> JAMA:79). In a study of heart attack victims, it was found that people who took high doses of niacin had an 11 percent lower death rate than those who did not. Niacin must be administered in high doses to be effective in lowering blood cholesterol. But because of the significant side effects of large doses of niacin, it should be taken only under a doctor's supervision. Some people, such as those with high blood pressure, diabetes, gout or ulcers, should not take niacin at all. The niacinamide form of the vitamin should not be used because it does not lower blood fats by a significant amount. Food sources for niacin include yeast, fish, poultry, liver, meat, whole-grain products (except corn which contains an inactive form of niacin), peanuts, potatoes, beans and mushrooms.

• Beginning at the age of two, children from families with a history of heart, circulation or cholesterol problems should begin cholesterol-reduced diets. If either of the child's parents has a high cholesterol level or if one of the child's parents or grandparents has suffered a heart attack before 60 years of age, the child's diet should be closely controlled. A low cholesterol diet will be healthy for the child, and will train the child to have good, lifelong dietary habits. It is much easier to raise a child on skim milk and low amounts of fried foods, cheese, eggs and ice cream than it is to try to change the diet of an adult. A strict diet is not necessary for the child unless serum cholesterol level is high. However, teaching moderation to children in high-risk families may prevent them from developing heart and artery disease in their lifetimes.

Cold Feet
Cold feet may be a result of poor circulation caused by clogged arteries, heart problems, or stress. Many people with diabetes, rheumatoid arthritis, collagen disease or lupus suffer from cold feet. Smokers often get cold feet because the effects of tar and nicotine in the tobacco cause the arteries to clog and cause poor circulation. If you suspect that your cold feet are related to a circulation problem, you should discuss it with your doctor.

Simple exercise is the best way to warm up cold

feet. Aerobic exercise, like walking, bicycling, swimming or jogging, is the best. With sustained aerobic exercise, the heart and blood vessels increase their tone. Circulation is improved, and, usually, the feet warm up. For an elderly person confined to bed or a chair, even rocking in a rocking chair can help improve circulation and warm up the extremities.

A warm or hot bath will raise body temperature and warm up the feet. If a bath is not practical, soak your feet in warm water. Placing a hot water bottle or an electric heating pad on the feet may also help. Do not get the water or heating pad too hot because the feet will not be sensitive, and you could burn yourself very easily.

Of course, wearing heavy socks or slippers is an easy way to keep the feet warm. Many people wear socks to bed because even blankets and comforters do not seem to keep their feet warm enough. Placing a blanket, quilt or afghan over the legs and feet while sitting is also effective. Many nursing home residents and people confined to a bed or a wheelchair use "lap quilts" to help keep their legs and feet comfortable.

Constipation
- To avoid constipation, increase your intake of

fiber by eating:

> Whole-grain cereals, rye crackers, bran, breads and flours made with whole-grains

> Fruits

> Vegetables. People who wish to maintain a high level of fiber in their diets should not peel their fruits and vegetables. Much of the fiber content of these foods is in their peels.

> Legumes are the vegetables with the best source of fiber. Legumes include peanuts, peas and beans. Vegetables that are from the root of the plant, like carrots and potatoes, are also good sources of natural fiber.

> Switch from white rice to brown rice to increase fiber content. Remember, what we call fiber today, is what our grandmothers used to call roughage. They knew, as we know now, that your diet must include enough roughage to aid in proper digestion and excretion of food. By the way, roughage turns to mush in the body after it absorbs water in the stomach.

• Drink more water. Adults should drink eight glasses of water each day. According to research on constipation by Lederle Laboratories, feces are 75 percent water. Hard feces found in constipation contain less water. A person must drink plenty of fluids each day to help in the excretion of soft stools.

• Get regular exercise. Lack of exercise is a common cause in constipation. Inactivity is one reason why constipation is prevalent among many older people.

• Constipation may be caused by certain prescription drugs. Many prescription drugs like antidepressants, pain relievers containing narcotics, diuretics, and drugs used to treat Parkinson's Disease can cause constipation. Some over-the-counter drugs like laxatives and antacids containing calcium and aluminum can also contribute to the problem of constipation.

• Physical or emotional stress can also add to constipation problems. During pregnancy, while traveling or during times of severe stress, be especially careful to eat plenty of fiber and drink lots of fluids.

• Avoid holding your breath when straining during a bowel movement, says Cardiac Alert newsletter. This "Valsalva Maneuver" counteracts the natural tendency to hold the breath during a bowel movement or when you are trying to lift, pull, push or move something. Many times, people hold their breath and groan while straining. Holding your breath during a bowel movement causes your blood pressure to skyrocket and puts additional pressure on your heart and arteries. Practice breathing in and out slowly and steadily during all bowel movements or any strenuous event.

Straining during a bowel movement may cause hemorrhoids and bowel problems. High-fiber diets help people avoid straining at stool.

• If you suffer from prolonged constipation, lasting over a week, see your doctor. Extended constipation could be a sign of a more serious illness, like cancer of the colon, irritable bowel syndrome or diverticular disease in the colon.

Croup

Croup can be a very frightening disorder for a young mother and the child. Usually the child has difficulty breathing, coughs, and may have a slight fever. The <u>American</u> <u>Medical</u> <u>Association's</u> <u>Handbook</u> <u>of</u> <u>First</u> <u>Aid</u> <u>and</u> <u>Emergency</u> <u>Care</u>, recommends that you try to calm the child first. The child and the parent both need to try to remain as calm as possible to keep croup under control. If it is a minor episode of croup (lips have not changed color, no fever, and the child responds well to calming), moist heat may help the child breathe properly. Take the child into the bathroom and close the door. Turn the hot water on in the tub or shower, but DO NOT put the child in the water. Stay in the closed room, with the moist heat, for about 20 to 30 minutes. The moist heat should help to open the child's breathing passages and return the breathing to normal, suggests the AMA. Do not put anything in the child's mouth because it may block the child's air passage.

Dental Problems

• Brushing your teeth after eating and flossing at least once each day are still the best ways to prevent dental problems. Besides brushing teeth and tongue after each meal, you should brush immediately after eating sugary candy or dried fruit, like raisins, prunes or figs. If you cannot brush, you may try eating certain cheeses or chewing sugar-free gum. Sweets that are allowed to stay in the mouth for long periods of time can cause cavities.

Research led by Charles Schachtete, Ph.D. at the University of Minnesota, revealed that some cheeses neutralize the acid formed by sweets and, thus, reduced the number of cavities. Only Swiss, Cheddar and Monterrey Jack cheese worked to stop sugar from "attacking" the teeth.

Other research has shown that chewing sugar-free gum helps reduce decay-causing acid. Sugar-free gum helps keep sugar from remaining on the teeth, which helps to reduce cavities.

• Avoid swimming pools with high chlorine levels. The Centers for Disease Control (CDC) in

Atlanta says that swimming in a pool with a high chlorine level can cause cavities because the water is so acidic. The acid will erode tooth enamel. For people with their own pools, the pH level should be kept at 7.2 or above, according to the CDC. In public pools, ask the lifeguard or pool manager about the pH level. If the public pool often has a low pH level and seems to be over-chlorinated, it may be better to find another pool!

• If you take antihistamines, drink plenty of fluids. People taking antihistamines, usually people with allergies, experience more tooth decay because the antihistamines dry up their saliva. The decrease in saliva will cause an increase in the number of cavities and gum problems, according to an article in <u>Family Circle</u> (7/8/86). <u>Consumer Reports</u> (October 1986) says that other types of drugs can cause dry mouth, which leads to tooth decay. Antidepressants, blood pressure reducers, tranquilizers and some ulcer drugs may also cause this unwanted side effect. People taking any of these drugs should brush their teeth more often and drink plenty of water or other sugar-free drinks to avoid an increase in dental problems. If you have a dry mouth or extensive tooth decay and are taking one of these medications, discuss the situation with your dentist and your doctor. Your doctor may want to switch to a similar medication that won't cause dry mouth.

• Bad habits can harm our teeth and gums, says the Academy of General Dentistry. To protect our teeth and gums, the Academy listed several common habits that we should avoid (from <u>Ladies Home Journal</u> February 1987):

> Do not chew hard objects, like popcorn kernels, ice, hard candy, pens and pencils. They can erode, break or damage teeth, crowns and fillings.

> Do not bite your fingernails (or toenails). Nails are hard substances that can damage the teeth and gums.

> Toothpicks may help get food out from between the teeth, but they should not be used as a wedge between the teeth. The root structure of the tooth can be severely damaged by an ordinary toothpick. If you want to massage your gums, use a Water Pik® or similar device, the rubber tip on the end of some toothbrushes, or special brushing aids available at your drug store.

> Do not suck on lemons or oranges. The strong acid from these fruits can harm the tooth's enamel and soften its root structure. Many athletes suck on lemons and oranges before a big race or competition. However, it would be better for them to drink orange juice or actually eat the fruit. Damage to the teeth occurs when the acid remains in the mouth for long periods of time.

> Avoid chewable vitamin C. Several dentists

claim that people who are taking vitamin C supplements in chewable form are destroying their tooth enamel. They suggest simply swallowing vitamin C if you wish to take supplements.

Also see: **Gum Disease.**

Depression

• Abnormal sleep patterns may cause depression in some people, according to Gerald W. Vogel in the Archives of General Psychiatry (March 1980). Normal sleep patterns include several stages of sleep leading to a very deep sleep involving Rapid Eye Movements, referred to as the REM stage. In Vogel's study at the Georgia Mental Health Institute, he discovered that severely depressed people usually experience more REM sleep. It usually occurs earlier in the night than in a non-depressed person. However, if the bedtime were changed to several hours later and the sleep pattern was mixed up, the patient's depression greatly improved. Unfortunately, changing the sleep patterns is only a temporary cure. If sleep becomes too irregular there is not a pattern to break and the person becomes depressed again. Some prescription drugs, like antidepressants, monoamine oxidase (MAO) inhibitors and tricyclics, also change the sleep pattern and help relieve depression.

• Inderal® and other beta-blocking drugs, prescribed to help lower high blood pressure, may cause depression, according to a study in the Journal of the American Medical Association (JAMA 255: 357-360). More than 20% of people taking beta-blockers eventually start taking antidepressant drugs, says Dr. Jerry Avorn of Harvard Medical School, who conducted the study. Dr. Avorn says this is the first study that confirmed the linkage between depression and beta-blockers, although many doctors have suspected a connection for several years. Many other prescription drugs, including sleeping pills and tranquilizers, can cause depression. If you suspect your medication is causing your depression, discuss it with your doctor. Never stop taking a prescribed drug without your doctor's consent.

• Unusual feelings of hunger and cravings for sweet food are experienced by about 50% of people taking drugs for depression, according to the journal Geriatrics (41:4). The report warns that everyone, espeically diabetics and people with high blood pressure should avoid overeating when they are on antidepressant drugs. The unusual cravings often cause people to eat more than normal and to gain weight. Being overweight is dangerous for everyone, but especially for those with high blood pressure or diabetes. The pangs of hunger and cravings for sweets seem to be side effects of antidepressant drugs that stop as soon as the drugs are discontinued, says the report. If you suspect that your prescription drugs are causing these side effects, discuss them with your doctor. Do NOT stop or change your medication without your physician's approval.

• John Crayton, M.D. at the University of Chicago, suggests that the food we eat may affect our moods. His tests indicate that wheat and milk can cause increased depression and irritability.

• Richard Wurtman, Ph.D., from Massachusetts Institute of Technology (MIT) reports that the amino acid, tyrosine, was helpful in treating depression. One woman that Dr. Wurtman treated found that her depression lifted while she was taking supplements, but returned within a week after the tyrosine supplements were stopped. Be careful! Quick acting substances may cause tolerance to develop and not be helpful in the long run. Tyrosine is found naturally in beans, seaweed, whole-grain products, green beans, aged beef, aged cheese, milk, yogurt and pickled herring.

Diabetes
• Massaging the site of an insulin injection can help get more of the medicine into a diabetic's

system, says <u>Modern</u> <u>Medicine</u> (52:122,43). For diabetics on insulin shots, the researchers recommend massaging the injection site for three minutes after the insulin injection. Dr. Richard S. Dillion of Bryn Mawr Hospital in Pennsylvania reports that more insulin will get into the person's system with this method. In two years of research with 26 diabetics, Dr. Dillion found that massaging improved the ability to maintain consistent blood sugar levels.

• Exercise may help improve a person's sensitivity to insulin, according to a study in the <u>Journal</u> <u>of</u> <u>the</u> <u>American</u> <u>Medical</u> <u>Association</u> (JAMA 252:645). Many diabetics over 60 years of age seem to lose their responsiveness to insulin treatment. As the insulin seems to lose its effectiveness, the incidence of heart and artery problems increases. A study at the Washington University School of Medicine in St. Louis showed that people over 60 who participated in regular exercise did not experience a lower response to the insulin. When exercise programs were started for diabetics over 60 who had already experienced a decrease in the insulin tolerance, their insulin sensitivity greatly improved. To retain sensitivity to insulin, older diabetics should exercise for at least 45 minutes, three times each week. The exercise could be walking, jogging, cycling, or using a treadmill. The researchers reported that more strenuous activity improved the response better than less strenuous exercise.

Your physician should be consulted before beginning any new physical activities. He can help outline a program suited to your needs that will begin with less strenuous exercises and gradually increase to more difficult ones.

Research at the Veterans Administration Medical Center in Birmingham, Alabama, has shown that inositol helps eliminate nerve pain associated with severe diabetes. Inositol is not considered to be a vitamin, so it does not have an official RDA (Recommended Daily Dietary Allowance) set by the U.S. government. However, inositol is generally recognized to have many vitamin-like qualities and is important in the functioning of the nervous system. The best food sources of inositol are organ meats, yeast, beans, (especially great northern beans), whole-grain products, peanuts and citrus fruits (especially grapefruit or orange juice) and fresh cantaloupe. Caffeine interferes with the body's use of inositol; so don't use any products that contain caffeine. Biotin, choline and vitamin E are needed for inositol to be used most effectively in the body.

• Diabetics and people with high blood pressure should avoid overeating when they are taking anti-depressant drugs. Unusual feelings of hunger and cravings for sweet food are experienced by about 50% of people taking drugs for depression, according to the journal <u>Geriatrics</u> (41:4). The unusual cravings often cause people to eat more than normal and gain weight. Being overweight is dangerous for everyone, but especially for diabetics. The pangs of hunger and cravings for sweets seem to be side effects of antidepressant drugs that stop as soon as the drugs are discontinued, says the report. If you suspect that your prescription drugs are causing these side effects, discuss them with your doctor. Do NOT stop or change your medication without your physician's approval.

Emphysema See: **Lung Diseases.**

Eye Problems
Reduced vision in the elderly is sometimes related to poor lighting in their homes, according to an article in <u>The Lancet</u> journal. Researchers at London's St. Bartholomew's Hospital discovered that many elderly people in their homes used only one-tenth of the light used in the hospital. When the elderly people added a small light with a 60-watt bulb to illuminate their homes, vision improved in 82% of the patients. Before loss of vision in the

elderly is assumed to be permanent, home lighting should be checked.

Fatigue

• People suffering from chronic fatigue should try wearing a pedometer, according to Dr. Peter J. Steincrohn. A pedometer is a small device that is worn to see how many miles a person walks. It is often used by people while hiking or walking for daily exercise. However, Dr. Steincrohn recommends wearing it to show how much walking people do in their daily routines. Many people, he believes, do far more walking than they realize. Often, people will go to their doctors complaining about constant fatigue. They will say and believe that they are inactive. By wearing a pedometer during a normal day's activities, people can gauge how much walking they are really doing. Using the pedometer, they can have an accurate count that may surprise them and their doctors. Once the number of miles in a regular day has been calculated by the pedometer, chronic fatigue can be reduced by cutting back in walking or activities that are excessive. Keep wearing the pedometer so you can judge if you are eliminating enough activity, the doctor suggests. Don't cut out activity that isn't excessive. Most people suffer from too little, not too much, exercise.

Dr. Steincrohn also recommends cold showers and short naps to help fight fatigue. Cold showers are more effective than hot showers or baths, he says. The cold water increases red and white blood corpuscles, lowers body temperature and increases the oxygen supply, which decreases the fatigued feeling. Warm or hot water will only raise the body temperature and increase fatigue, Dr. Steincrohn explains.

Men suffering from fatigue should try wearing a girdle around their waist, suggests Dr. Steincrohn. This doctor believes, and has supporting testimonies, that wearing a girdle (often called an abdominal support) helps ease the strain on the heart. Supporting the abdominal muscles helps increase circulation. To ask a man to wear a girdle may sound utterly ridiculous . . . but once most men with weak abdominal muscles try it for a week, they realize that they are less fatigued, says Dr. Steincrohn. Wearing a girdle that provides support of the "pot belly", seems to be an easy and inexpensive method to reduce fatigue in men.

• Chronic fatigue may be caused by a nutritional deficiency, says Dr. D. Lindsay Berkson of the Nutrition Revolution in California. If someone does not digest his food properly, the body does not get the nutrition from the food, and the person becomes tired. Dr. Berkson recommends that if you suffer from chronic fatigue, severe abdominal pain, and a lack of ability to concentrate, you should consult a physician about possible digestive problems.

Food Allergies

Food allergies can cause immediate or delayed reactions like hives, swelling, headaches, eczema (an itchy scaling, swelling and crusting of the skin), worsening of asthma, tight throat, vomiting, wheezing, shortness of breath, stomach cramps, aching joints, diarrhea, bloating or water retention, upset stomach, runny nose, stuffy nose, tiredness, inability to concentrate, skin reactions like itchiness or rash, belching, constipation, swelling of the face, itchy eyes, canker sores in the mouth, inflammation around the lips, dizziness, ear problems, difficulty in urination, hoarseness, strong mood swings or emotional disturbances. Sometimes food allergies cause severe reactions, like an irregular heartbeat, a drop in blood pressure or anaphylactic shock, that require emergency medical treatment.

• Almost any food will cause reactions in some people, but there are some foods that have been identified as being the most troublesome. Here are some of the foods associated with allergic reactions:

> Most often: corn, eggs, fish, cow's milk, nuts, seafood, wheat.

> Often: alcohol, berries, buckwheat, cane sugar, chocolate, citrus fruit, coconut, coffee, MSG (monosodium glutamate), mustard, oranges, peanut butter, peas, pork, potatoes, soy sauce (and other soy products), strawberries, tomatoes, yeast.

> Sometimes: apples, bananas, beef, carrots, celery, cheese, cherries, chicken, cottonseed, food-coloring dyes, food-flavoring additives, food preservatives, garlic, green beans, lettuce, melons, mushrooms, oats, onions, plums, pepper, prunes, spices, spinach, vitamins, water impurities often found in household tap water, chlorinated water and softened water.

• Most food allergies are not obvious. They are usually caused by our everyday foods and have less apparent, but nagging symptoms. Allergic reactions to food can be delayed or immediate. Sometimes people will feel sick while eating the food, but more likely, the reaction will take several hours, or even days.

• Eating isn't the only way to get an allergic reaction to food. Sometimes, the aroma of a cooking food can trigger the reaction.

• Beware of how food is prepared. Some foods may be tolerated only after they're cooked, since cooking breaks down some of the food's substances. However, in some people the opposite can be true — they may be able to eat the food raw, but react to it when it is cooked. Some foods are more likely to cause allergies if they are fully ripe. For example, the more ripe tomatoes are, the more likely that they will cause an allergic reaction.

• Avoid groups of related foods. For example, if you are allergic to peanuts, you should be careful about eating other foods of the same family like soybeans, peas and legumes.

• Watch the additives, even in your fruits and vegetables. Pesticides (to kill insects and rodents), herbicides (to kill weeds) and fungicides (to stop the growth of mold) are used when growing and storing foods, but washing or peeling won't remove all of them. These chemicals go right through the food and actually become part of the food during the growth of the plants. Fruits that grow on trees receive the most chemicals. Perhaps the only way to overcome the pesticides, herbicides and fungicides in your food is to grow your own food, or purchase it from health food stores or local co-ops where you know how the food was raised, transported and stored.

• Eating in restaurants can be very difficult for allergy-prone individuals because all of the ingredients in menu items are not identified. If you think something on the menu might cause problems, the waiter may be able to find out the names of the ingredients, but some chefs may be reluctant to reveal their "secret" recipes. If you have a serious allergy, you may want to patronize a few favorite restaurants where you can discuss the ingredients with the chef, or you may decide to avoid restaurant cuisine.

• Once allergies are identified, trying to avoid the annoying foods is a problem. Food labels are hard to understand, but it is extremely important that people with allergies read the labels and eat only what they can. Remember, labels can be tricky because even simple food labels can be misleading. For example, vegetable oil could be from corn, peanut, sunflower, olive or another vegetable! Here are some label tips for people with specific allergies:

> Milk allergy — Watch for caseinate, lactose or whey because all are milk based additives. Many "nondairy" creamers contain these additives. In recipes, substitute water, soy milk, or fruit juice for cow's milk.

> Egg allergy — Avoid vitellin, ovotellin, livetin, ovomucin and albumin.

> Wheat allergy — Beware of flour, wheat flour, wheat starch, gluten flour, cracked wheat, malt, graham flour, monosodium glutamate

(MSG), hydrolyzed vegetable protein, and durum flour.

> Corn allergy — Don't eat dextrose (corn sugar), cornstarch, corn oil, corn syrup, glucose, dextrin, dextrimaltose, or fructose. Avoid most table salt because it contains corn sugar. Many cough syrups, cough drops, lozenges, pills, tablets and suppositories contain corn. Vitamin and mineral supplements also can be corn-based.

• Addiction to Food — Some people have an allergic addiction to some foods, usually very common ones. They must eat a certain food to avoid having "withdrawal" symptoms. Their addiction actually masks the allergic reaction to the food. Many people who are "allergic-addictive" crave foods, or eat certain foods at the same time every day. They may call themselves "chocolate-holics" or "foodaholics".

Some obese people and some alcoholics fall into this category. They are actually allergic to the food or drinks they crave or react abnormally to them, yet they must eat them to avoid a withdrawal reaction. Eating the offending food may give them a "high" or a positive feeling. To break the food addiction cycle, the person should completely avoid the offending food for at least five days. However, as an alcoholic must avoid all alcohol, the "foodaholic" must continue to avoid offending foods to completely overcome the addiction.

Food Poisoning

The risk of food poisoning can be lowered by following these few suggestions from <u>Prevention</u> magazine (4/86).

• Do not allow hot food to cool down in a window or on a counter-top. As the food cools down, it will be in the optimal temperature range for the growth of harmful bacteria. Food ready to be stored should be placed immediately into the refrigerator while it is still hot. Large amounts of hot food, like a pot of stew, can cause other food in the refrigerator to heat up, so food should be separated into smaller containers.

• Thaw frozen meat in the refrigerator. Frozen meat that is thawed on the counter-top can develop harmful toxins from bacterial decomposition that may not be destroyed by cooking. If you plan ahead and allow time to defrost the meat in the refrigerator, it will not get warm enough to spoil.

• Store foods below 40°F. Between 40° and 120°, bacteria will flourish. At picnics and outings, do not allow the food to sit out or get warm. Try to eat within at most two hours after the food leaves the refrigerator.

• Botulism is a potentially fatal disease; thirty

percent of people who get botulism die. Home-canned vegetables should ALWAYS be boiled before eating to avoid botulism from improper canning. Do not even taste them before they are completely cooked.

• Do not eat food from a can with swollen ends or a jar with a swollen lid. Do not eat food that looks, smells, or tastes funny. Jams, jellies or fruit juices should not be used if they taste fermented. Foods with mold, odd coloring or foam should also be discarded. If you know that food is bad, try to dispose of it in a place where no other humans or animals could get to it.

• Do not eat eggs that are dirty or cracked. Egg shells should always be washed, even if they do not appear to be dirty. Wash the shells, even if you are going to use the raw egg for baking.

• Do not eat raw foods except for unspoiled, fresh vegetables or drink raw milk. Oysters, sushi, steak tartare, unpasteurized milk and other raw foods have caused several serious outbreaks of food poisoning.

• About 40% of commercially-sold raw chicken has salmonella, a bacterium that causes severe food poisoning, according to research by Iowa State University. Salmonella and campylobacter are commonly found in raw meat and food that is not cooked thoroughly. Poultry, meat and seafood should be cooked to an internal temperature of 165°F to kill all bacteria. When reheating leftovers, they should also be cooked to 165°.

• When cooking a turkey, don't put the stuffing inside the bird until you are ready to pop it into the oven after thoroughly scrubbing the inside of the turkey with salt. If you stuff the turkey the night before and put it in the refrigerator, the stuffing will stay warm because the cold cannot penetrate through the turkey. Bacteria could grow in the stuffing, and the whole turkey could be ruined. The safest way to prepare dressing is to bake or cook your stuffing separately. However, if you prefer to cook it inside the turkey, scrub the inside of the turkey with salt and stuff the turkey at the last possible moment.

• When you cut or prepare raw meat on a cutting board, clean the cutting board and utensils with soap and hot water before using them for other food. Wash your hands thoroughly before working with other food. The germs from raw meat can stay on the cutting board, the utensils and your hands.

• Washing your utensils in a dishwasher will help remove any contamination. If cleaning by hand, you may want to rinse the utensils and dishes with a chlorine bleach and water solution to sterilize them.

• Do not place cooked meat back on the plate you

had stored it on when it was raw unless you clean the plate thoroughly. The juices and germs left over from raw meat can contaminate cooked meat. This is especially important to remember when barbecuing.

• Do not taste food, especially meat or fish dishes, before it is thoroughly cooked.

• Do not taste food with a dirty or used spoon. Your saliva can contaminate the food. Always use a clean spoon for tasting.

• Always wash your hands before preparing food. It is especially important to wash your hands after smoking, going to the bathroom, sneezing, blowing your nose, biting your nails or putting your fingers in your mouth or nose.

• Do not prepare food if you are sick, have boils, severe acne, or an infected cut on your hands.

Foot Problems

Diabetics and people with circulation problems or nerve damage in the feet are especially prone to foot problems. Amputation may be necessary if sores in such people aren't treated quickly. Here are some tips on good foot care from <u>Women's</u> <u>Day</u> magazine (7/8/86) and the <u>Better</u> <u>Health</u> newsletter (10/86):

• Wash your feet daily, but do not soak them for

long periods of time. Soaking may cause them to dry out. If you shower, you should wash your feet separately, in a basin of warm, sudsy water. If you have nerve damage in your feet, be sure to check the water temperature before you put your feet into the basin or tub.

• Dry your feet carefully. Be gentle, yet thorough.

• If you have problems with foot odor, excessive perspiring of the feet or fungus growth on the feet, you may want to sprinkle medicated or plain foot powder on your feet after drying them. Powdering between the toes and on the soles of your feet is best. Use as little powder as possible. If the powder clumps, you have used too much.

• If you have problems with dry skin on your feet, you may want to moisturize them at least once a week. Use a water-based moisturizer or petroleum jelly. To avoid possible fungus infections, don't put moisturizer around your toenails or between your toes. Apply the moisturizer just before going to bed, and put on a pair of socks. The socks will keep the moisturizer on your feet and not on the bed linens.

• Inspect your feet daily if you are in a high risk category for serious foot problems. Let your doctor know if you develop an ingrown toenail, blister, bunion, bruise or a sore that seems slow to heal. People at high risk should not use harsh preparations to treat their foot problems. Gentle massaging with a soft washcloth is acceptable. See your doctor or podiatrist (a foot specialist) as soon as possible when problems occur.

• Never break or lance a blister. Don't tear off any "loose" skin. You should cleanse the area including the loose skin. Clean loose skin serves as a natural bandage. It will protect the problem area from infection and help speed the healing process.

• Trim or file your toenails straight across. Curving the nail will increase the incidence of ingrown toenails.

• Don't cut your toenails shorter than the end of the toe. The shorter the nail is cut, the more chance of developing an ingrown toenail.

• Using an emery board, file each nail until it is smooth.

• Buy and wear shoes that fit properly. If the shoes do not fit properly in the store, do not allow the salesman to "stretch" them or alter them. Don't buy them if they don't fit the first time you put them on.

• Buy shoes in the afternoon or evening to get a proper fit. During the day your feet swell slightly. If you buy your shoes in the morning, your feet may be smaller than usual, and the shoes will not fit later on.

• Buy shoes that give your toes plenty of breathing room. There should be at least a quarter of an inch between your longest toe and the end of the shoe. Avoid pointed shoes because they don't give your toes enough room.

• If you suffer from ingrown toenails, you should not buy sandals or shoes without a toe cover. Ingrown toenails can be aggravated if they are banged or stubbed. Be sure to wear shoes that will protect your toes and toenails.

• Wear high heels as little as possible. They are acceptable for short periods of time, but do not wear them if you must do a lot of standing or walking.

• Buy shoes that are made of natural materials or fabrics. Vinyl, plastic and other man-made materials will not allow the feet to breathe. Without proper ventilation, infections, blisters and foot odor can flourish.

• If you are elderly or have difficulty walking, try to buy shoes with soles that grip the floor. Many soles have special ridges in them to help reduce slipping and falling.

• For the best support and comfort, buy shoes with flexible soles that will cushion your feet.

• When you buy a new pair of shoes, break them in slowly. If you are buying shoes for a specific event, try to buy them at least two weeks early.

Wear the shoes around the house for an hour each day. Breaking in shoes gradually will help prevent blisters and soreness from occurring.

• Keep your shoes in good repair. Don't allow the heels to get worn or the soles to wear unevenly.

• Do not wear slippers when you need the support of a pair of shoes.

• If you suffer from dry, cracked feet, DO NOT go barefoot. Otherwise, going barefoot is good only on soft surfaces like sand, grass and soft dirt. Do not even go barefoot for long periods of time in your own home. Without any protection, your feet could lose natural oils and be damaged.

• Don't wear socks that have seams or darning in them. These irregular surfaces may cause blisters or irritation of the feet.

• Natural fibers like cotton and wool are better than socks made from synthetic materials which don't absorb perspiration well.

• Wear clean socks. If your feet perspire a lot, try changing your socks twice a day.

• Don't wear socks that are tight at the top. They may reduce blood circulation to the foot.

Gout

Gout is the only form of arthritis that, in most cases, can definitely be controlled by a proper diet that is low in meat and other foods that contain purines. At one time, gout was considered to be a disease of the rich. Many wealthy people, who overindulged in rich food, suffered from gout. However, gout can affect anyone.

Gouty arthritis is a metabolic disorder affecting the body's whole system, not just individual joints. It is caused by an over-accumulation of uric acid in the body. If left untreated, gout can lead to death from kidney disease, high blood pressure or coronary heart disease.

• Because it is a metabolic disorder, it usually can be controlled by eating a low purine or purine-free diet. After the first onset of gout, limiting purine intake can usually control future attacks and prevent joint damage. Purines are present in many foods. The following foods should be avoided to help control the symptoms of gout.

> Foods containing high amounts of purine: anchovies, bacon, beef, brains, calf tongue, carp, chicken soup, cod fish, consommé soup, duck, fish roe, fowl, goose, gravy, halibut, heart, herring, kidney (beef), lentils, liver, liver sausage, meat extracts, meat soup, partridge, perch, pheasant, pigeon, pike, pork, quail, rabbit, sardines (in oil), shell fish, sweetbreads, trout, turkey, veal, venison.

> Foods containing moderate amounts of purine: asparagus, beans, bluefish, bran, bran flakes,

cauliflower, chicken, crab, cracked wheat, eel, fish, graham bread, graham crackers, graham porridge, ham, kidney beans, lima beans, malt breakfast food, mushrooms, mutton, navy beans, oatmeal, oysters, peas, puffed wheat, rolled wheat, rye bread, rye krisp, salmon, shad, shredded wheat, spinach, tripe, tuna fish, wheatcakes, whitefish, wholegrain products.

> All meat, game and fish contain purines. Therefore, any meat should be eaten in small portions.

> Alcohol should be avoided since it aggravates gout.

> Condiments, spices, seasonings of all types, concentrated sweets, rich pastries and fried foods should be restricted in the diet.

> Fats should be limited because they interfere with the removal of uric acid from the body.

> Drink plenty of fluids. Two quarts of fluids each day will help reduce the concentration of uric acid in the blood and help keep uric acid crystals from forming on the joints.

Gum Disease

Prevention is the best way to fight most gum disease which causes more loss of teeth than cavities. Trench mouth, an infectious disease of the mouth and gums that also causes bad breath and a metallic taste in the mouth, can be treated or prevented. Emory University's Dwight Weathers, D.D.S. suggests that many people, who are under a great deal of stress and do not eat properly, suffer from trench mouth. After medical treatment has cleared up the infection, good oral hygiene, a diet featuring fresh vegetables and fruits, and learning to manage stress will help keep this gum disease from recurring.

The first stage of common periodontal gum disease, called gingivitis, occurs in most people as they age and affects the gum line at the base of the teeth. The advanced stage of this disease is known as periodontitis. Periodontal gum disease can lead to the loss of many or all of your teeth, but it can be prevented.

Here are some suggestions to reduce the risk of gum problems:

> Brush your teeth and tongue after every meal. Brush immediately after eating sugary candy or dried fruit.

> Use a toothbrush with soft bristles — hard bristles can damage the gums and the enamel on your teeth.

> Use a salt, soda, or salt and soda solution instead of commercial toothpaste, recommends Dr. Paul Keyes at the National Institute of Dental

Research.

> If you use a commercial toothpaste, use a tartar control formula.

> Floss at least once daily.

> Massage your gums by using a Water Pik® or similar device, the rubber tip on the end of some toothbrushes, or special brushing aids.

> Reduce your intake of sugary foods and candies or eliminate them entirely from your diet.

> Have your teeth professionally cleaned at least twice a year.

> Daily rinsing with a new prescription mouthwash will kill the bacteria that cause gum disease. The active ingredient in the mouthwash is chlorhexidine gluconate. The mouthwash is approved by the Food and Drug Administration (FDA) and the American Dental Association (ADA). It is sold by prescription only under the brand name Peridex®. It is thought to be a breakthrough in preventing gum disease for people who cannot floss (due to physical handicaps) and people with low production of saliva.

> Vitamin C may help prevent gum disease, according to research by Dr. Robert Jacobs at the Western Human Nutrition Research Center.

• Some problems or habits increase the severity of gum disease. Most of these problems alone will not cause gum disease, according to the FDA

Consumer (18:7). However, since many conditions can worsen gum disease, proper dental hygiene is especially important if you:

> Smoke or chew tobacco.

> Grind or clench your teeth (often as a reaction to stress).

> Have teeth that are not aligned properly.

> Receive poor nutrition.

> Have diabetes.

> Wear dentures that do not fit correctly.

> Are pregnant.

> Bite your nails, chew popcorn kernels, or chew ice cubes.

> Take oral contraceptives, anti-cancer drugs, steroids or anti-epilepsy drugs.

If you are highly susceptible to gum disease, Dr. Dwight Weathers recommends eating foods that are high in vitamin A. He says that vitamin A can help strengthen gum tissue and that a deficiency of vitamin A can lead to gum problems. However, Dr. Weathers warns that vitamin A is toxic in high doses. Do not take excessive vitamin A supplements, but increase your intake of foods rich in vitamin A. Natural sources of vitamin A or carotene, which a healthy body converts into vitamin A, include eggs, whole milk products, broccoli, spinach and other green, leafy vegetables, sweet potatoes, carrots, pumpkins, and squash.

Also see: **Dental Problems.**

Hair Problems

• According to Dr. Kenneth A. Arndt, Associate Professor of Dermatology at Beth Israel Hospital, some prescription drugs and these traumatic events can cause a change in the body's production of hair:

> childbirth
> major surgery
> a high fever
> a lengthy or severe illness
> great emotional stress
> a strict weight-loss diet
> a large loss of blood

However, within several months hair production should resume.

Some problems cause permanent hair loss, Dr. Arndt explained in the <u>Harvard</u> <u>Medical</u> <u>School</u> <u>Health</u> <u>Letter</u>. Cancer, a severe deficiency of iron, thyroid disease, and diabetes may cause irreversible hair loss.

• To make the most of the hair you have, Janis Buller of Vidal Sassoon in Beverly Hills, suggests:

> Layering the hair. Hair cut in short layers will appear to be fuller.

> Use conditioners on your hair to help keep it looking full.

97

> Wearing a beard will give the impression of having more hair on the head.

> Keep hair fashionably short. Short, well-kept hair and a beard will give the illusion of more hair.

> Men with bald spots should not keep some hair long and try to lay it over the bald spot. It will call attention to the lack of hair, and it looks worse than the bald spot.

> Rinses and shampoos containing protein may help rebuild hair that has been physically damaged.

• To avoid unnecessary damage to your hair, limit:

> Exposure to ultraviolet rays (from sun or tanning booths).

> Exposure to heat (from curling irons, hot curlers and blow dryers).

> Combing, brushing, shampooing, teasing, perming, coloring, tinting or using hair sprays, mousses and gels.

Headaches

Headaches can be annoying and debilitating. To treat them effectively, it is important to know what kind of headache you are experiencing. According to Howard D. Hurland, M.D., author of Quick Headache Relief Without Drugs, these are the things you should know about your headaches:

> When did the headaches begin? If they began suddenly, during a certain season of the year or while you were under some personal stress, it may it easy to pinpoint the type of headache you are experiencing. For example, a seasonal headache starting in the fall or spring could be an allergic reaction to pollen. Headaches that start during times of unusual stress could be tension headaches. These usually occur at the same time of day and are fairly constant.

> What type of pain is the headache causing? Some people have short bursts of sharp pain while others have a dull aching pain.

> Where is the pain? Is the pain centered in one area or one side of the head? If so, you may have a migraine headache.

> Have the headaches progressed in severity? Does it seem like the headaches are getting worse and worse? Headaches that start suddenly and continue to get more severe could be a warning sign of a brain tumor. If you get this kind of headache, you should contact your doctor at once.

> When do they occur? Is there a pattern to when you have them? For example, if you have them about four hours after eating, but they go away when you eat again, you may be suffering from low blood sugar. Just eating smaller, more frequent meals may help prevent this type of

headache. Other headaches frequently are caused by eating certain foods. If you can keep track of when the headaches occur and how long they last, you may discover some food allergies that are causing the headaches. Are headaches a reaction to your emotions? Do you suffer from more headaches when you are angry or under stress?

> Is any other part of your body affected by your headaches? Problems with your sight, watery eyes or blurring associated with your headache may show that you are suffering from migraines.

> What other things seem to occur when you experience your headaches? Many prescription and over-the-counter drugs can cause headaches as a side effect. Do you have headaches only when on a certain type of medication? Do they occur when you are outside? Do they occur when you are under fluorescent lights? Do flashing lights bother you? Are they related to your menstrual cycle? Any circumstance that seems to trigger your headaches may provide clues to preventing the headaches.

> Has anyone else in your family, like your mother or father, suffered from a similar type of headache? Migraine headaches may be an inherited condition.

> Does anything help relieve the pain? If you take one aspirin or lie down and the pain goes away, it may be a very different kind of headache

than one that requires a lot of painkillers.

> Does anything seem to make the headache worse? If you lie down and the headache seems to get worse, it could be a migraine headache. Headaches that are caused by brain tumors seem to get worse when the neck is constricted or during a sudden move, like a sneeze

• People with migraine headaches should avoid food containing tyramine. Tyramine dilates the blood vessels and contributes to many headaches. Avoid certain foods in the following groups because they contain high concentrations of tyramine:

> meat/fish — chicken livers, sausages, pickled herring, dried fish and beef.

> dairy — aged cheese, sour cream and yogurt.

> alcohol — red wine, champagne, sherry, beer, ale, Riesling and sauterne wines.

> vegetables — sauerkraut and fava beans (broad Italian beans).

> flavorings — chocolate, soy sauce, vanilla and yeast.

Nitrites are also known to cause certain types of headaches. Watch for nitrite or nitrate additives on product package labeling. Be sure to avoid:

> hot dogs.

> bacon.

> sausage.

> pepperoni.
> salami.
> ham.
> all processed luncheon meats.
> all cured meats.

• Many people have severe headaches after eating food containing monosodium glutamate (MSG). MSG is often used in Chinese cooking, and these headaches and associated symptoms have been referred to as the Chinese Restaurant Syndrome. If you suffer from headaches after eating Chinese food, stop eating at Chinese restaurants or discuss with the chef the availability of MSG-free foods. MSG is also found in some meat tenderizers and prepared frozen dinners — be sure to read the labels.

• Migraine headaches may be helped by resting quietly in a dark room for a couple of hours. Place a cool washcloth on your forehead. Make sure the cloth has been rinsed in cold water and wrung out. Or just sprinkle some cold water on your face before you lie down.

• Dr. Seymour Diamond, director of the National Migraine Foundation, suggests placing an ice pack against your forehead or wherever the pain is coming from. According to a recent study at the Diamond Headache Clinic, over 80 percent of migraine sufferers decided the cold pack treatment helped reduce their headaches. Because a migraine headache is caused by the swelling of blood vessels, an ice pack may cause the blood vessels to return to a normal size, and the pain will cease, Diamond explains. For the best effect, he recommends placing the ice pack directly on the head and lying down for 30 minutes.

• If it's not possible to lie down, try holding your hands under cold running water at a wash basin. This often provides some relief by causing the blood vessels in the hands to constrict, thereby affecting the body's vascular (blood vessel) system.

• Tension headaches may be helped by a simple massage of the scalp, neck and jaw area. Tension headaches are those with a dull, steady pain. Usually they are caused by tension or eyestrain. Relaxation techniques, like taking a warm bath or listening to soft, calming music, may help. Refrain from all alcohol.

• Caffeine may provide relief from some headaches but cause headaches in other people! According to Harold Gelb, D.M.D. in <u>Killing Pain Without Prescription,</u> drinking one or two cups of coffee may help constrict the blood vessels and reduce some people's headaches. However, constricting the blood vessels can cause headaches in other people, and withdrawing from habitual use of caffeine often causes headaches for a few days. Before you try coffee, tea, or other caffeine-containing products for headache relief, be sure you know if you are sensitive to caffeine.

Heart Problems

Smoking seems to increase the risk of a heart attack, even if you don't have hardening of the arteries, according to new research from Emory University in Atlanta. In a group of people under 60 years old who did not have hardening of the arteries but suffered heart attacks, over 71% had a history of smoking. Only 48 people were involved in the study, so the results are only preliminary. However, it seems to be an additional reason to quit smoking.

• A high white blood cell count increases a person's risk of having heart disease. According to a recent study at the University of Minnesota, people with a high white blood cell (WBC) count have a higher risk of developing heart disease. The abnormally high level of white blood cells can cause damage to the artery walls, says Dr. Richard Grimm, Jr. Smoking, another risk factor in heart disease, is extremely dangerous when combined with a high white blood cell count, Dr. Grimm warned.

• Heavy coffee drinkers may increase their risk

of heart disease by as much as three times the risk of non-coffee drinkers, according to a study at Johns Hopkins Medical Institute in Baltimore. The researchers found that men who drank five or more cups of coffee daily were 2.8 times as likely to develop coronary artery (or heart) disease as normal. The study, published in the New England Journal of Medicine, included 1,130 males. It seems that an occasional cup of coffee is all right, but heavy coffee drinking should be avoided. The more coffee you drink, the more you are increasing your risk of coronary artery disease, angina and a sudden heart attack, the researchers concluded.

• Veins in your neck that suddenly begin to stand out, could be a warning sign of heart problems. According to Dr. Frank Field in Family Circle magazine (10/1/86) , the veins in your neck can fill with blood when the heart is failing. Many heart specialists will examine the neck as part of their routine check-ups. If you notice a change in the veins of your neck, contact your doctor.

• Avoid holding your breath when straining, says Cardiac Alert newsletter. This "Valsalva Maneuver" is the natural tendency to hold your breath during a bowel movement, while exercising or when you are trying to lift, pull, push or move something. Many times, people hold their breath while straining. The Valsalva Maneuver is especially common during weight-lifting. However, holding your breath during these strenuous times causes your blood pressure to skyrocket and puts additional pressure on your heart and arteries.

Practice breathing in and out slowly and steadily. Consciously breathe during any strenuous activity. Then, when lifting or moving something, be sure to have enough people or support to properly help you move the object.

Avoid all straining during bowel movements. As well as increasing your blood pressure, the strain may cause hemorrhoids and bowel problems. High fiber diets help people avoid straining at stool.

• Be very careful in the mornings. A recent study by Harvard University researchers showed that most sudden cardiac deaths occur between 6:00 a.m. and noon. After reviewing over 2,000 death certificates of heart attack victims, the researchers published their findings in the journal, <u>Circulation</u>. Doctors are not exactly sure what factors increase the risk of an early morning death. Perhaps the normal rise in blood pressure that is experienced in the morning as we awake or increased production of blood platelets which may cause blood to clot may be among the causes. Previous victims of heart attack or people with heart problems should take extra care before noon.

• Beware of sudden spurts of strenuous activity. Moderate, medically supervised, regular exercise, started gradually, may help in living with or recovering from certain heart problems. However, sudden spurts of activity, weekend exercise, or exercise taken just because you "feel like" exercising is NOT good for your heart and arteries, says Dr. Peter J. Steincrohn. It is a paradox that many studies show that regular, sustained aerobic exercise strengthens the heart and helps circulation, while other studies show that sudden, unaccustomed bursts of exercise can lead to heart attacks in susceptible people.

Before you shower after exercising, cool down, warns Dr. John Cantwell in the American Medical Journal (252:429). Cantwell, the team doctor for the Atlanta Braves baseball club, says that showering too soon after exercising can cause spasms in your arteries or a sharp decrease in blood pressure. Exercise causes a fall in blood pressure because the blood tends to collect in the legs after exercising, he explains. If you take a hot or warm shower while in this condition, the hot water can dilate the blood vessels and create an even greater drop in blood pressure. On the other hand, a cold shower can raise blood pressure and place a sudden strain on the heart. This could cause some arteries to go into spasms, explains the doctor. To avoid any bad effects, Dr. Cantwell says that after exercising, you should completely cool down before heading for the showers.

• People receiving digitalis or other heart medication should not take calcium ascorbate (a vitamin C formulation) since irregular heartbeats may occur.

• When niacin (vitamin B3) is taeken in high doses, it has been shown to reduce the amount of cholesterol in the blood (<u>Journal</u> <u>of</u> <u>the</u> <u>American</u> <u>Medical Association</u> JAMA:79). In a study of heart attack victims, it was found that people who took high doses of niacin had an 11% lower death rate than those who did not. Niacin must be administered in high doses to be effective against heart disease and cholesterol. But, because of the significant side effects of large doses of niacin, it should be taken only under a doctor's supervision. Some people, such as those with high blood pressure, diabetes, gout or ulcers, should not take niacin at all. The niacinamide form of the vitamin should not be used because it does not lower blood fats by a significant amount. Food sources for niacin include yeast, fish, poultry, liver, meat, whole-grain products (except corn which contains an inactive form of niacin), peanuts, potatoes, beans and mushrooms.

For some heart patients, an aspirin a day can

reduce the chance of having another heart attack, the Food and Drug Administration (FDA) says. One aspirin tablet per day can cut heart attacks by 20%, for most people who have already had heart attacks, to as much as 50%, in men who have unstable angina. According to the FDA, for patients who had had a previous heart attack, an aspirin a day reduced the chance of having another heart attack or of dying of a heart attack, by about one-fifth. Aspirin is not a substitute for other preventative therapies for heart attacks, cautions FDA commissioner Frank E. Young, M.D. He advises that patients consult their physicians before starting daily aspirin as therapy. The studies don't show whether aspirin would be effective in preventing heart attacks in healthy people, just in people with history of heart attacks or angina.

Avoid areas of air pollution. Ozone, sulfur dioxide, nitrogen dioxide, cigarette smoke, carbon monoxide, hydrocarbons, nitrogen oxide and photochemical substances are air pollutants that can worsen heart problems.

Living at high altitudes may not be as harmful to the heart as has been thought. In the past, doctors thought that high altitudes caused heart problems. However, new research by the American Heart Association shows that the opposite may be true. James K. Alexander, M.D. of Baylor College of

Medicine in Houston, participated in the study called Operation Everest Two. Over a 40-day span, seven men were put into a low-pressure chamber that simulated the effects of 29,000 feet altitude. Dr. Alexander said they were surprised to discover that the heart actually seemed to do better at high altitude! In spite of this study, sudden changes to high altitudes should be avoided, and people with severe heart disease may be helped by moving to low altitudes. Ask your physician for his advice.

Recovering from a heart attack can be difficult, especially when a spouse is worried about your every move. Researchers at Stanford University tried an experiment that allowed the spouse to participate in the physical therapy of the heart attack victim. Not only did they watch the activities, they felt compelled to perform the same treadmill stress tests, side-by-side with their spouses. According to an article in Body Bulletin, the loving spouses could see and experience the physical activity and stress of the treadmill. Once they knew how the heart attack victim had endured the exercise, they didn't worry about them as much at home during their recovery. They encouraged their partners and were more tolerant of their activities. By having a spouse's support, recovery was less stressful and a little easier for the heart attack victim.

See also: **Cholesterol Reduction.**

Heartburn

Some prescription and over-the-counter drugs, including aspirin and ibuprofen, can cause heartburn. Estrogens can weaken the muscle that keeps stomach acids in the stomach. Any woman taking estrogens, including estrogens in birth control pills, or a pregnant woman who has a natural increase in estrogen production is more likely to suffer from heartburn, according to the <u>Harvard</u> <u>Medical</u> <u>School</u> <u>Health</u> <u>Letter</u>. If you are taking any medicine, discuss your heartburn problem with your doctor. Your doctor may want to choose an alternative drug or reduce or eliminate any drugs that might be causing the heartburn.

See also: **Indigestion, Hiatus Hernia.**

Hiatus Hernia

Hiatus (or hiatal) hernia occurs when the sphincter muscle at the opening of the stomach from the esophagus becomes separated from the surrounding tissues. The muscle is intended to keep food and acid in the stomach from being regurgitated up into the esophagus. When the sphincter muscle is torn or cannot do its job effectively, acids irritate the esophagus and throat. Pain, commonly called heartburn, is often experienced. Women over 40 years old are at the highest risk of getting hiatus hernia. Severe hiatus hernia may have to be repaired by surgery, but natural methods of treatment often can make heartburn go away.

• Hiatus hernia can be caused by using tobacco. Quit using cigarettes, pipes, cigars, chewing tobacco, or snuff.

• Heartburn during the night can be caused by eating too near the time you lie down to sleep. Doctors recommend that people should not eat large suppers and not eat within three hours of bedtime.

• If you are regularly bothered by indigestion in the night, try raising the head of your bed by six to ten inches. Use wooden blocks or bricks under the legs of the bed. This should create enough difference in the level of your head and your stomach so that acid will not flow up out of the stomach.

• During the day, do not lie down if you are bothered by heartburn. Sitting or standing helps to keep the stomach acids in the stomach.

• Hiatus hernia or heartburn can be caused or aggravated by obesity. Losing weight, especially if you're fat around the stomach, may help. Consult your doctor for diet and exercise suggestions.

• Avoid bending over. Bending puts pressure on your abdomen, which can aggravate the heartburn.

- Do not wear tight clothes, girdles, or belts.
- Chocolate, peppermint, tobacco of any kind, aspirin, coffee, tea, alcohol, fried foods, tomato products, onion, garlic, citrus fruits and juices, spicy or fatty foods can all cause problems and should be avoided.
- Constipation can cause problems. Increasing the amount of fiber in the diet may eliminate constipation and reduce the additional pressure on the stomach.
- During pregnancy, the additional pressure on the abdominal muscle can cause heartburn. The discomfort it brings can temporarily be treated with antacids. The types of antacids which coat the stomach and which are dispensed in liquid form are most effective in relieving heartburn caused by pregnancy.
- Develop good eating habits. Eat slowly by putting your knife and fork down between bites. This will reduce the amount of air you swallow with each bite and will slow down your eating.
- To further reduce the amount of air you swallow, don't talk while you are eating, don't drink carbonated soft drinks, and don't chew gum.
- Eat small meals. If you can eat six small meals rather than three large meals, you should experience less heartburn.

Hyperactivity

Hyperactivity in children is often treated with drugs. However, doctors writing in the <u>Harvard Medical School Health Letter</u> believe that behavior modification may be just as effective as drugs. Behavior modification involves changing the way a child behaves by setting goals and giving rewards for good behavior. The doctors warn that this requires more patience and understanding than most parents or teachers are willing to give.

Some doctors recommend changing the diet of hyperactive children by eliminating food additives and/or refined sugar. Some children seem to respond to the change in diet perhaps because they have an allergic reaction to the food additives or sugar. Dietary changes probably help only a small percentage of hyperactive children.

Be reasonable and discerning before labeling a child as hyperactive or accepting such a label from teachers. Young children and pre-teens are easily distracted and naturally have much higher energy levels than adults.

Impotence

According to the journal <u>Urology</u> (April 1986), smoking is the biggest contributing factor in impotence. In a study of over 1,000 men suffering from impotence, 78% were smokers. Smoking, and the clogging of the arteries that it brings, was more strongly associated with impotence than high blood pressure, age or diabetes, all possible contributing factors. A man's ability to achieve an erection is based on a good blood supply to the penis. When the blood supply to the penis is reduced, so is the chance of achieving an erection.

A similar study published in The Lancet confirms these conclusions. The Lancet research showed that men who have several risk factors for hardening of the arteries tend to have problems with impotence. Smoking is a major risk factor in hardening of the arteries and cardiovascular problems. Men who smoke and suffer from impotence should quit smoking.

Indigestion

• Sleeping on a water bed can aggravate indigestion, according to new research at the University of Rochester in New York State. Sensations of floating and the pull of gravity may caused indigestion, says the report. To reduce the moving sensations, water beds with baffles that stop the free flow of water are recommended. When reclining, be sure that your head is not lower than your stomach, or stomach acid may escape and create indigestion.

• Camomile tea, made from the camomile herb, is an old folk remedy for indigestion that is worth trying, says Varro E. Tyler, Ph.D. Boil half an ounce of camomile in 1 1/2 cups of water. Let it sit for at least ten minutes to get the most out of the herb, he suggests. Take a few sips of the tea, several times each day as needed. Dr. Tyler is the dean of the Schools of Pharmacy, Nursing and Health Sciences at Purdue University.

Another herb recommended by Dr. Tyler for indigestion is capsicum. Capsicum is commonly known as chili pepper. While some may think that chili pepper causes more indigestion than it helps, Dr. Tyler disagrees. Only a very small amount of capsicum, less than 60 milligrams, is necessary to help relieve an upset stomach, he says. Capsicum can also be used to relieve stomach pain, flatulence, diarrhea, cramps and muscle aches, according to Dr. Tyler.

• Aspirin, ibuprofen, over-the-counter pain-relievers, and vitamin C in the form of ascorbic acid, can cause an upset stomach. To avoid indigestion after taking them:

> Always take aspirin, ibuprofen or ascorbic acid only after eating.

> Take them with milk or water. Never take them with an acidic juice, citrus fruit or alcohol.

> Do not take aspirin and vitamin C together.

This can increase the risk and severity of indigestion.

> Vitamin C in the form of ascorbic acid should always be taken with food or with a large amount of water and an antacid.

> If aspirin and ibuprofen continue to cause indigestion, consider switching to an enteric-coated brand of aspirin or ibuprofen, or change to acetaminophen. Enteric-coating allows the drugs to be released in the bowel instead of the stomach, which will reduce or eliminate stomach irritation. However, the enteric-coated drug will take longer to become effective.

Infertility

• Proper vaginal lubrication is often an important element in conception. Petroleum jelly can kill sperm. Water or saliva may hamper the sperm in their travels through the vagina, say researchers at Emory University in Atlanta. They recommend egg whites as the perfect lubricant while trying to conceive. Dr. Andrew Toledo, a gynecologist at Emory's Infertility Clinic, says that egg whites actually help the sperm swim toward the egg. Since egg whites are protein and so are the sperm, the egg whites make it easier for the sperm to travel, Dr. Toledo explains.

Using egg whites is still in an experimental stage. However, dozens of children have been born in Atlanta to parents who had fertility problems until they used egg whites as their lubricant. Since egg whites are not expensive, are easy to obtain and are a natural lubricant, Dr. Toledo hopes they will help many more couples to conceive.

• Even small increases in temperature in a man's groin can lower sperm counts and reduce fertility in men. According to an article in Prevention magazine, a recent study by Dr. Richard J. Paulson at the University of Southern California School of Medicine tested sperm counts in volunteers after a relaxing hour in a hot tub. Dr. Paulson believes that this is the first scientific experiment to test the effect of heat on sperm. Within 36 hours of the time in the tub, the sperm could not penetrate an ovum. The number of sperm dropped, according to the study. It took 7 weeks for the sperm count to return to normal.

Men who are trying to have children should not overheat the groin area. They should avoid hot tubs, steam baths, long hot baths, and jockey shorts. Boxer shorts are preferred because jockey shorts hold too much heat in the groin.

• If a woman is taking fertility drugs, she should avoid taking vitamin C supplements. Vitamin C may block some of the activity of the fertility drugs. Vitamin C itself may help increase fertility, but it should be avoided, if possible, while on fertility drugs.

Insomnia

• Commonly prescribed drugs, stimulants and stressful lifestyles can cause insomnia. Here are some of the usual causes of sleeplessness, cited by the Harvard Medical School Health Letter:

> Lack of routine sleeping habits, especially inconsistent bedtimes or waking times.

> An emotional crisis, such as work-related problems, loss of money or marital problems.

> Being overaroused. Worrying about tomorrow's activities or planning events while trying to sleep is not productive. Perfectionists often suffer from this type of insomnia because they keep reviewing details in their mind, rather than relaxing and preparing for sleep.

> Lack of exercise or daily activities. Unemployment or physical infirmities may limit daily activities.

> Caffeine. Avoid all sources including coffee, tea, chocolate, soft drinks, and some prescription and over-the-counter drugs. Ask your pharmacist for a complete list of drugs that contain caffeine.

> Developing a tolerance to sleeping pills.

> Alcohol. It is common to awaken in the middle of the night after drinking alcohol.

> Over-the-counter diet pills (most contain stimulants).

> Certain prescription drugs including:
—asthma drugs.
—blood-pressure reducing drugs.
—heart-rhythm regulating drugs (anti-arrhythmics).
—hormones, like estrogen, progestin, oral contraceptives, and adrenal hormones.
—steroids.
—levodopa and other drugs used to treat Parkinson's disease.

> Being bored or lacking a purpose in life.

> Depression.

> Naps taken during the day.

> Snoring or other breathing problems that interrupt normal sleep.

> Nervous system diseases affecting the brain, spinal cord or nerves.

> Severe pain, fever or itching that disturbs sleep.

> Gland problems involving the thyroid gland, parathyroid gland, ovaries, testes, pituitary gland, adrenal gland or the pancreas.

> Illegal drugs like marijuana or cocaine.

• Fresh air in the bedroom may help alleviate

insomnia. Opening the windows wide for about 10 minutes, then leaving them open about an inch, can provide a good supply of oxygen and fresh air for the night's sleep. A stuffy room may inhibit your ability to sleep, according to Dr. Charles Wolfe, Jr. of the Sleep Disorder Center in Chicago, Illinois.

Creating your personal perfect environment for sleeping can be helpful, according to the Mayo Clinic Health Letter. Fresh air, a cool room temperature, total darkness, quietness, and clean bedsheets may help you get a good night's sleep.

• If you are in a situation where complete silence is impossible to achieve, try masking the sounds. A small air-conditioning unit, a fan, a stereo or a radio set at low volume may block out annoying sounds and create a monotonous environment for sleeping.

• Don't get physically or mentally excited in the evenings. Don't exercise at night. Avoid sex just before bedtime if it leaves you in an excited state. However, some people find sex a release. They may find it easier to sleep right after sex.

• A warm bath may be helpful to induce sleep. Dr. Peter J. Steincrohn says warm or hot water will raise the body temperature and increase tiredness. Warm water also aids in reducing tension and helps the mind to concentrate on peaceful things, which should make it easier to fall asleep after the bath.

• Progressive relaxation is a simple technique that may also help. Starting with the muscles in your toes, each muscle group is tensed and relaxed several times. By the time you work your way up through your toes, feet, calves, thighs, stomach, arms, to your neck, you should be very relaxed.

• A glass of warm milk may be helpful. This is an old folk remedy that seems to have scientific basis to help insomnia. Dr. Ernest Hartmann in Boston has shown that L-tryptophan, an amino acid found abundantly in milk, helps people get to sleep easily. According to Dr. Hartmann's research, L-tryptophan stimulates the production of serotonin which is involved in the brain's sleep process. L-tryptophan supplements are available in some health food stores. However, we do not recommend taking these supplements regularly because other research has shown that L-tryptophan supplements may speed the aging process. At this time, it seems that drinking warm milk is the best way to get the benefit of this amino acid. L-tryptophan is also found in other dairy products, as well as in bananas, tuna, sardines (with bones), soybeans and turkey.

Taking the herb, hops, may help lull you to sleep, says Varro E. Tyler, Ph.D., dean of the Schools of Pharmacy, Nursing and Health Sciences at Purdue University. Hops are known for their role in making beer, but they also have a sedative effect, he explains. A few years ago, people who harvested hops were found to become sleepy and tired after just a short time at work in the fields. Their behavior led to the discovery of hops as a sedative, according to Dr. Tyler. For the best sedative effect, Dr. Tyler suggests putting some hops in a muslin or cloth bag and using the bag as a pillow.

• Eat a lot of carbohydrates at your evening meal or as the last food you eat before going to bed. Eating meals composed mainly of carbohydrates may help people relax and feel drowsy, according to research at Texas Tech University. Psychology professor Dr. Bonnie Spring measured the difference between the effects of carbohydrate and protein meals in 184 people. Proteins made the people feel tense, but carbohydrates relaxed the men and made the women feel drowsy.

Kidney Disease
Using large amounts of pain killers, especially aspirin and the banned painkiller, phenacetin, may lead to kidney damage, according to the Harvard Medical School Health Letter.

Arthritics and women who are chronic headache sufferers often use aspirin excessively. Once people stop taking the pain-killers, the kidneys may be able to function properly again. However, the newsletter warns that heavy use of aspirin could lead to permanent kidney damage, requiring the person to use kidney dialysis or seek a kidney transplant.

Kidney Stones
• Changes in diet can help many people avoid kidney stones, which tend to recur in susceptible people. To prevent most, but not all, kidney stones:
> Drink eight glasses of water or fluids each day.
> Avoid carbonated soft drinks. A research study from the University of Florida published in the Journal of Chronic Diseases (38:11) indicated that carbonated cola drinks containing sugar were the top drink used by men who suffered from kidney stones. Milk, water, tea, beer and coffee were also tested as the primary beverage for several groups, but they did not seem to be associated with a higher incidence of kidney stones. The consumption of excessive phosphorus, which is present in large quantities in carbonated soft drinks, is known to drive calcium from the bones. This mineral imbalance may play a role in kidney stone formation.
> Eat a diet low in protein.
> Empty the bladder frequently and completely.
> Get adequate amounts of pyridoxine (vitamin B6) and magnesium in your diet or as supplements.

Magnesium and pyridoxine have been used to limit or stop calcium oxalate clumping, which is a major cause of kidney stones. Taking supplements of 25 milligrams of pyridoxine per day may help prevent kidney stone occurrence or recurrence.

> People who know they have a tendency to produce kidney stones may want to avoid large doses of vitamin C. High doses of vitamin C may cause high levels of uric acid in the blood. Some studies, according to <u>Vitamin Side Effects Revealed</u>, indicate that large doses of vitamin C can create conditions which, theoretically, might increase the rate of oxalate kidney or urinary tract stone formation. However, other studies indicate that people who take large doses of vitamin C do not have an increase in the rate of stone formation.

• For people who form kidney stones from calcium and oxalate, Dr. Steven Kanig, a medical professor at the University of New Mexico, recommends:

> Reducing the amount of calcium in the diet. Calcium is found in dairy products, leafy, green vegetables, salmon and sardines.

Calcium is generally a beneficial mineral, so this advice isn't good for everyone, only stone formers.

> Reducing the amount of oxalate in the diet. Oxalate is a mineral found in spinach and other green, leafy vegetables, tea and chocolate.

Leg Pains

People suffering from leg pains should try wearing a pedometer, according to Dr. Peter J. Steincrohn. A pedometer is a small device that is worn to see how many miles a person walks. It is sometimes used by people while hiking or walking for daily exercise. However, Dr. Steincrohn recommends using it to measure how much walking people actually do in their daily routines. Many people, he believes, do far more than they realize. Often a person will go to her doctor complaining about leg pains. She will say and believe that she is inactive.

By wearing a pedometer during a normal day's activities, people can gauge how much walking they are really doing. Using the pedometer, they can have an accurate count that may surprise them and their doctors. Once the number of miles in a regular day has been calculated by the pedometer, if it's excessive, leg pains can be helped by reducing walking and increasing the time the legs are raised.

Caution! Daily activity like walking usually is a great health benefit. Don't reduce your activity unless it's excessive or unless your doctor recommends it.

Lung Diseases

To lower your risk of diseases that obstruct your

breathing, don't smoke. Lung diseases like bronchitis and emphysema are often associated with smoking or other forms of air pollution. Some lung damage associated with smoking will never be repaired once a person quits, but quitting may prevent the disease from progressing further.

• Avoid areas of high levels of pollution. Pollution over certain cities, like Denver, London and Los Angeles, has been known to contain sulfur and nitrous dioxide which can aggravate cases of asthma, bronchitis and emphysema. Chemical air pollution, present in certain occupational settings, can also contribute to lung diseases, according to the <u>Harvard Medical School Health Letter</u>. Welding fumes, cotton dust, some vapors from the production of plastic, gases from smelters and even aerosol sprays used in the home contribute to lung diseases, says the Harvard publication.

• Drink plenty of water, at least eight glasses a day, to help keep the throat clear.

Breathing exercises may also help restore easier breathing. Check with your doctor or, perhaps, see an inhalation therapist.

Menopause
Many emotional problems, claimed to be caused by the "hormonal imbalance" of menopause, may

have a more direct cause. According to doctors writing in <u>Family</u> <u>Circle</u> magazine (11/5/85), sometimes the physical problems of menopause contribute to the emotional problems. For example, hot flashes during the night can cause an interruption of sleep and consequent bad moods or depression the next day. Such mood changes are actually caused by the lack of sleep, not a hormonal change. Therefore, treating the physical problems associated with menopause, like insomnia, hot flashes and sweating help lessen the emotional swings.

Morning Sickness

Morning sickness may seem like "all day and night sickness" for some pregnant women. Nausea and vomiting, associated with pregnancy, do not always occur in the morning. They can occur at any time. They can cause a pregnant woman to lose the nutritious food that both she and her baby need. Women who are pregnant for the first time, especially young women, are more likely to suffer from morning sickness.

• Here are a few suggestions that may help calm a queasy stomach:

> First of all, DO NOT smoke. Not only does smoking add to the frequency of nausea in pregnant

women, smoking harms the unborn child. Please, for the sake of your baby, do not smoke during pregnancy.

> Try eating a few crackers, melba toast, dry toast or unbuttered popcorn when you feel sick.

> Do not eat fried food, butter, margarine or anything greasy.

> Eat several small meals throughout the day, rather than eating any large meals. Small meals will be easier to digest, and you won't get a full or uncomfortable feeling.

> If you are bothered by nausea in the morning, try eating something light before you get out of bed. A couple of crackers may be all it takes to ease that sick feeling.

Motion Sickness

Eating a couple of green olives may help prevent motion sickness. Excess saliva and stomach acid are produced during motion sickness, which adds to the feeling of nausea. Green olives contain tannins. Tannins, Dr. Cecil Hart from Northwestern University Medical School explains, help reduce the production of saliva and stomach acid and, therefore, may prevent nausea.

Nail Problems

• White spots on the fingernails, split nails, and soft nails that peel are often caused by a diet that is low in zinc. The mineral zinc is found naturally in liver, seafood, dairy products, meat, eggs and whole-grain products.

• Ridges or pits in nails may be caused by psoriasis, a common skin condition. Psoriasis can also cause toenails and fingernails to lose their shine or become discolored. Also see: **Psoriasis.**

• Brittle nails may be caused by a deficiency of iron, overuse of nail polish or nail polish remover, or exposure to harsh chemicals or detergents, according to Paula Blake, R.N. in Bestways magazine. To improve the condition of the nails:

> Take better care of your hands and feet. Don't expose them to chemicals or detergents. Use rubber gloves when washing dishes or doing major cleaning.

> Eliminate nail polish. Allow your nails to "breathe".

> Try an iron supplement. According to a study done in Sheffield, England, many women with brittle nails simply have a low iron level. Taking an iron supplement will often improve nails as well as energy levels!

> People with low thyroid levels often have brittle nails. If you have low energy and suspect a

problem with your thyroid, discuss it with your doctor as soon as possible.

> Discoloration of the nails can be related to several different internal problems like breathing disorders, tuberculosis, cancer and diabetes, especially in the elderly. If your toenails are yellow and your feet have small red patches on them, contact your doctor for a glucose tolerance test to see if you have diabetes.

> People with nails that break, crack, peel or chip may not be properly digesting their food, according to research by Johnathan Wright, M.D.

Dr. Wright suggests that poor nails may be a sign that the stomach is not producing enough acid. Without sufficient acid, the body may not properly absorb the nutrition from the food that is eaten. Dr. Wright suggests taking betaine hydrochloride or glutamic hydrochloride with pepsin supplements to increase levels of stomach acid. However, this solution will have to be continued indefinitely if the stomach will not produce enough acid on its own.

Check with your doctor for his approval and to make sure that you really suffer from low levels of stomach acid before trying this remedy.

Nerve Pain
Nerve pain, or neuritis, may be alleviated or

prevented by a diet high in inositol. Research at the Veterans Administration Medical Center in Birmingham, Alabama, has shown that inositol helps eliminate nerve pain associated with severe diabetes. Inositol is not officially considered to be a vitamin because it can be made inside the body of a healthy adult, so it does not have an official RDA (Recommended Daily Dietary Allowance) set by the U.S. Government. However, inositol is generally recognized to have many vitamin-like qualities and is important in functioning of the nervous system.

The best food sources of inositol are organ meats, yeast, beans, (especially great northern beans), whole-grain products, peanuts and citrus fruits (especially grapefruit or orange juice, and fresh cantaloupe). Caffeine interferes with the body's use of inositol, so don't use any products that contain caffeine. Biotin, choline and vitamin E are needed for inositol to be used most effectively in the body.

Nightmares

Nightmares can be physically as well as psychologically disturbing. They are usually caused by stress, anxiety, terror or even the things we eat and drink. Don't worry if you suffer from an occasional nightmare. They are a normal response to stress and worry.

• Nightmares can be caused by an unusual strain on the emotions, like a crisis, a scary movie, or a disturbing book or experience. If you are prone to get nightmares, don't watch or read horror stories or any intense adventures just before bedtime.

• Nightmares can start after a difficult time like a death in the family or a serious accident. Such nightmares should not be a concern unless they continue for more than a few weeks.

• Avoid alcohol. Excessive use of alcohol or complete withdrawal from alcohol can cause nightmares.

• Learn to manage stress. Discussing your stressful problems with a friend or a professional counselor may subdue the nightmares.

• Some prescription drugs can cause nightmares as a side effect. Nightmares can also occur when you stop taking sleeping pills. If you start suffering from nightmares after you start taking a new prescription drug, check with your doctor or pharmacist.

• Nightmares are quite common with a high fever or illness.

• Some people find that eating certain foods or eating too close to bedtime will give them nightmares. Don't eat within four hours of going to bed, and don't eat heavy meals in the evening. If you have a nightmare, closely review the foods you ate and the things you did the day before the nightmare. If you have another nightmare, see if you can pinpoint a pattern and eliminate the behavior that preceded it. For example, if eating pizza gives you nightmares, you may want to give up pizza.

• If a child suffers a nightmare, giving comfort is most important. Comfort the child and allow him to relax and fall back asleep. Sometimes this is best achieved by quiet singing, hugging, patting or telling a calming story. Don't ask the child who's upset to describe his dream at that moment. Try to change the subject by putting a calm or happy picture in the child's mind. Try recalling a happy scene that the child can remember. If the child is old enough, you may want to talk about the nightmare the next day.

Osteoporosis

Osteoporosis is a serious weakening and loss of bone mass that usually affects women after menopause, although men and younger women also can suffer from it. The trace mineral manganese may be an important element in preventing osteoporosis. Manganese is necessary in bone and cartilage formation. People with a deficiency of manganese suffer from poor growth of bone and cartilage.

According to an article in <u>Bestways</u> magazine, basketball star, Bill Walton developed osteoporosis even though he was getting plenty of calcium, magnesium and B-vitamins. However, Walton's manganese level was nonexistent. Walton's bones got stronger with manganese supplementation. Walton was treated with manganese by his physician, Dr. Saltman, after research by Dr. Saltman revealed that the bones of rats who were put on a manganese-free diet became very brittle.

• One problem in fighting osteoporosis is that calcium, an essential mineral in the development of strong bones, reduces the availability of usable manganese in the body. Many women who are trying to prevent osteoporosis are consuming foods and supplements that are rich in calcium. By doing this, they may thus be depleting their manganese levels. Natural sources of manganese are whole-grain products, fruits (especially bananas), vegetables (especially legumes), liver, other organ meats and eggs.

• Lifelong observance of preventative measures is necessary to reduce the risks of osteoporosis later in life. Prevention of osteoporosis may be helped by:

< Adequate calcium intake. If possible, try to get plenty of calcium naturally through your diet. Dairy products (even low-fat varieties), leafy,

green vegetables (like broccoli, turnip or mustard greens and kale), salmon and sardines are high in calcium. Do not take calcium supplements unless you discuss it with your doctor. If you or your family has a history of kidney stones, taking extra calcium could be dangerous.

> Adequate vitamin D and vitamin E.

> Adequate magnesium, molybdenum and manganese, essential minerals.

> Weight-bearing exercise.

> Estrogen replacement therapy — the most effective treatment to prevent osteoporosis for women who have low levels of estrogen during or after menopause or complete hysterectomy.

> Not smoking.

> Reducing the amounts of caffeine, alcohol, salt, carbonated soft drinks and excessive protein or meat in your diet.

Pain

• Take pain-relieving drugs while standing up for fastest relief of pain. According to research published in the Clinical Pharmacology and Therapeutics journal, drugs start to relieve pain faster when you are standing, than if you are sitting or lying down. Common pain-killing drugs that are available over-the-counter are aspirin, acetaminophen and ibuprofen.

• Dr. Samuel Seltzer of Temple University has discovered that tryptophan supplements help relieve chronic head and neck pain. For tryptophan to work, Dr. Seltzer recommends a diet low in protein (about 10% of calories), low in fats (about 10% of calories) and high in complex carbohydrates (the remaining 80% of calories). In his study, relief from pain occurred in four to six weeks. Tryptophan is naturally found in turkey, beef, peanuts, bananas, pineapple, figs, dates, processed cheese and milk.

Panic Attacks

• Most people have experienced a small anxiety attack. Maybe it was while speaking in public, playing at a piano recital, or taking that first trip in an airplane. Anxiety is a natural reaction to the stress of specific events.

However, panic attacks sometimes occur without a specific event that is frightening or threatening. They may occur during the middle of the night, in a crowd of people, or even when walking down the street. The attack can be so strong that you can't think about anything else. You may be immobilized.

Panic attacks can be associated with deep-seated

worries or fears, maybe the fear of failing, frustration at not being perfect, or a feeling that you are no longer in control of your destiny.

Many people feel that they are having a heart attack, are dying or going crazy when they experience a panic attack.

Most attacks last between 5 to 30 minutes. If you experience four panic attacks within four months, you are suffering from a panic disorder and should get medical help, says the American Psychiatric Association. There are certain drugs that can help block panic attacks.

• The physical symptoms that accompany a panic attack may be the most frightening part of the experience. According to Reid Wilson, Ph.D., author of Don't Panic: Taking Control of Anxiety Attacks, these are some of the symptoms:

> heart palpitations
> feelings of suffocation
> sensations of choking
> tightening of the chest
> rapid breathing (hyperventilation)
> lightheadedness
> dizziness
> dry mouth
> sweating
> hot or cold flashes
> cold or clammy hands

> frequent urination
> backaches or neckaches
> twitches
> crying spurts
> shakiness
> disorientation or confusion
• Learn how to control and prevent panic attacks. Here are some practical suggestions that may be helpful:
> Use relaxation techniques.
> Learn to manage the stress in your life.
> Slow down your breathing. Practice breathing in very slowly to a count of 5. Then let your breath out to another count of 5. Slow breathing can relieve the heart palpitations. It can restore your carbon dioxide level, which may be low after rapid breathing. This will reduce lightheadedness, dizziness and tingling sensations.
> Try to focus on the task you are working on. If you can shift your thought to the task at hand, you may calm down.
• Dr. Reid Wilson recommends concentrating on being a "calm observer" of the situation. He found that many people can stop a panic attack when they visualize stepping outside themselves and observing the panic attack from a distance. Wilson suggests that you should try to look at the situation in a calm and rational manner to avoid increasing the

severity of the attack.

> Recognize that you will return to normal. Acknowledge that the attack is temporary, and you may overcome it sooner.

It is good to have an examination by your physician to ensure that a panic attack wasn't caused by another medical problem, such as too much thyroid hormone.

> An overactive thyroid gland can cause feelings of tension and apprehension resembling a panic attack. An overactive thyroid is usually accompanied by weight loss and eye problems. It should be treated by a doctor.

Pregnancy

• Pregnant women should not handle cat litter. A parasitic infection called toxoplasmosis can be transmitted by contaminated cat feces and may seriously injure the unborn child.

Dr. Kathryn Schrotenboer, a columnist for Family Circle magazine, suggests that a pregnant woman does not have to get rid of her cat if her vet agrees that the cat is not contaminated with the infection. However, Schrotenboer does recommend that women not change or touch the cat's litter box while they are pregnant. After contact with their cats, they should wash their hands thoroughly.

Pregnant women should also avoid eating raw meat dishes. Raw meat, like steak tartar or fillet American, can also transmit toxoplasmosis.

• A pregnant woman is more likely to suffer from heartburn or indigestion, according to the <u>Harvard Medical School Health Letter</u>, because of her natural increase in estrogen production. Among other things, estrogen affects the acid level in the stomach.

See also: **Indigestion.**

Premenstrual Syndrome (PMS)

• Swollen breasts, quick changes in emotions, fluid retention and other problems are associated with the end of the menstrual cycle. Most women experience some discomforts prior to menstruation, but some women suffer symptoms so severe that their normal activities and abilities are disrupted. Usually, if the symptoms are severe and continue for several days toward the end of each menstrual cycle, the woman is considered to suffer from PMS or premenstrual syndrome.

• Some doctors recommend that the first step in the treatment of PMS is for the woman to chart her menstrual cycle for at least three periods. All the symptoms need to be carefully recorded including severity, the day they started and the length of time they continued. Sometimes, a woman will discover that her symptoms last for only a few days, although they are so bad that it seems much longer. In this case, a more hopeful picture emerges. She will find that getting through two or three days is tolerable, knowing that the problem will soon end. However, when the chart shows severe symptoms for several days, the woman and her doctor should work to lessen the symptoms.

To make a chart, start with "day one" as the first day of your period. Across the top of the page, write in the date of the month, parallel to the day of your cycle. Down the left side of the page, write in the symptoms you usually experience during the month. These could include water retention, headaches, back pain, sore breasts, depression, weight gain, anxiety, irritability, arthritis, dizziness, tiredness, insomnia, cravings for sweets, salty foods or any other foods.

Mark the days of menstruation with an X. Fill in each day where a symptom occurs, noting the severity of the problem. If the problem is present but not aggravating, put an "L" for light. If it is severe enough to interfere with your regular activities, put an "M" for moderate. If the problem causes you to completely stop your normal activities, put an "H" for heavy. Keep track of your symptoms for about three cycles, then visit your gynecologist to work together on this problem.

• Many common problems can get worse during a woman's menstrual cycle, and these should be considered before PMS is thought to be the problem. The severity of arthritis, asthma, migraine headaches, depression, and blood sugar levels is sometimes increased during the premenstrual time in the cycle because of the normal fluctuation in hormone levels..

• Regular daily exercise may help reduce the tiredness associated with PMS. Exercise helps increase the amount of natural painkillers produced within the body. Exercise improves circulation. It may help reduce blood pressure. The person who exercises develops a sense of control over her body. Exercise also gives a woman a time each day when she is doing something for herself. As well as being physically rewarding, it provides a break from the regular stresses and strains.

• To combat the depression and irritability caused by PMS, doctors recommend eating four to six small meals, rather than three regular meals. Small, frequent meals will help regulate blood sugar levels in the body and help even out mood changes. Eating good foods, such as fruits, vegetables, whole-grain products and beans, will provide a healthful intake of nutrients. Mood swings and fluctuating blood sugar levels may also be helped by eating a little cheese or a small handful of nuts between meals. Avoid caffeine and alcohol.

• Fulfilling a food craving can cause fluid retention and mood swings. Eating salty foods, like potato chips, contributes to fluid retention. Craving and eating sweet foods can increase changes in moods and emotions. To help prevent PMS problems, it is best to cut down or eliminate salty or sweetened foods during the two weeks prior to menstruation. Eating a naturally sweet fruit may help fill the craving while providing good nutrition.

Psoriasis

• Psoriasis cannot be cured, but it can be treated by special skin cleansers, ointments, soaps, oils and shampoos. The exact cause of psoriasis is not known. Psoriasis is usually found as itchy pink or red spots with a characteristic silver scaling.

To treat common psoriasis, most doctors recommend over-the-counter creams and ointments containing coal tar derivatives. The skin must be kept clean, but not overly dry, to reduce flare-ups.

Here are tips to help prevent psoriasis flare-ups:

• Avoid aggravating the skin. Sunburn, other burns, cuts, poison oak or poison ivy can irritate the skin and increase the severity of psoriasis.

• Even though sunburn can aggravate psoriasis, regular, moderate exposure to sunlight helps clear up some cases of psoriasis. According to Consumer Guide®'s <u>Medical</u> <u>Symptoms</u> <u>and</u> <u>Treatments</u>, regular sunlight or controlled exposure to a sunlamp helps reduce psoriasis.

• Recognize that other factors, besides direct skin irritation, can affect this skin condition. Seasonal changes in weather can cause psoriasis to get worse. Some infections, like strep throat or respiratory infections, can increase its severity. In some people, stress can trigger a flare-up of psoriasis.

• Some prescription drugs, including beta blockers used for high blood pressure, lithium and chloroquine, can cause psoriasis flare-ups as a side effect.

Senility

• Senility is not something that naturally occurs just "due to old age". Most cases of senility are caused by Alzheimer's disease or damage to the brain caused by strokes. Senility from these causes is irreversible.

However, many types of false senility can be reversed if the cause of the senility is discovered. Gallstones, undiagnosed infections, drugs, depression, dehydration, vitamin deficiency, and heart disease can all cause reversible cases of senility.

• According to the <u>Harvard</u> <u>Medical</u> <u>School</u> <u>Health</u> <u>Letter</u>, misuse of prescription and non-prescription drugs is the number one cause of false senility. People on continuous medication often:

> Forget whether or not they have taken their pills.

> Forget to take their medicine at the proper times.

> Have several different prescriptions which have been prescribed by various specialists who do not know about the other prescriptions.

> Take over-the-counter medicines and vitamins without considering possible interactions with their prescription drugs.

• The following suggestions, including some from the <u>Journal</u> <u>of</u> <u>the</u> <u>American</u> <u>Medical</u> <u>Association</u> (JAMA), can help prevent senility symptoms caused by drugs:

> Inform your doctor(s) and pharmacist(s) of any medication you are already taking, including all prescription drugs, daily vitamin or mineral supplements and any non-prescription drugs like aspirin, acetaminophen, ibuprofen, cold medicines and laxatives that you take regularly. Many drugs interact with each other. Some drugs can lose or gain potency or cause serious side effects if they are

taken together.

> Use only one pharmacist, preferably one who has a computer for spotting possible drug interactions from the prescriptions he fills for each customer. Ask him to keep track of all prescriptions and to alert you and your doctors to any possible problems. Be sure this pharmacist also knows about any regular non-prescription drugs that you use.

> Keep a written record of any side effects you may experience while taking prescription drugs, and report them to your doctor. Loss of memory may be a specific side effect of a drug you are taking. If you can tell your doctor about side effects you have noticed, perhaps another drug without those side effects could be prescribed.

> Do not drink alcohol while taking any medication, prescription or over-the-counter, unless you have your doctor's approval. Alcohol may cause serious interactions with some drugs or increase their side effects or cause senility-like symptoms.

> If you have a complex timetable to take your drugs, or if you must take several different drugs, make a checklist so you can be sure what drugs you should take and when. Then check them off daily as you take them.

> Try to keep each prescription in the original container that the pharmacist supplies. The

container will protect the pills and give you the name of the drug and the daily schedule for taking the drug. Do NOT use containers with different compartments for each day unless your doctor agrees. Storing different drugs together in the same container can create chemical reactions and changes. Also, when drugs are combined in the same container, you could easily mistake one pill for another.

> Always follow the label instructions. There are good reasons why some medicine is to be taken with food, needs to be refrigerated or shaken well before using. If you don't follow these instructions, your medicine may be useless or even harmful to you. If the instructions are not clear, ask your doctor or pharmacist. Have them give you all instructions in writing, so you won't have to depend on your memory.

> Never take drugs prescribed for someone else. Drugs are prescribed on the basis of other drugs being taken, one's age, weight, health history and other factors. Exchanging medicine is extremely dangerous.

> Take ALL of your prescribed medicine, unless your doctor tells you otherwise. Just because you feel better doesn't mean you are completely well. Some medicine is prescribed to prevent problems, like high blood pressure, so you must take it as

prescribed, no matter how well you feel. If you really believe that the drug is no longer helping you, discuss it with your doctor. NEVER stop taking a prescription without your doctor's approval.

• Depression that is not recognized or diagnosed is the second leading cause of reversible senility, explains the <u>Harvard</u> <u>Medical</u> <u>School</u> <u>Health</u> <u>Letter</u>. Many times, symptoms of senility, such as loss of memory and deterioration of mental capabilities, are just shrugged off as "old age". If depression is not treated, the symptoms of senility will continue, and the person will get worse. However, if depression is properly diagnosed, therapy could restore the person to good health.

Also see: **Depression**.

• An untreated physical disease can also cause symptoms of senility. If relatives dismiss senility as simply a result of "old age," a serious physical problem, like an infection, a blood clot or even alcoholism, could go untreated.

• Keeping mentally active will help avoid loss of memory. Reading, playing games, joining a discussion or tour group, becoming a volunteer, or any number of other mentally challenging activities will help maintain mental clarity.

Skin Problems

• Rub your hands together briskly before applying make-up, moisturizer, cleansers or fresheners
to the face. Vera Brown, a skin care specialist on
the TV program, <u>Hour Magazine</u>, says that this
provides warmth to the face and helps improve the
circulation. When cleansing the skin, you should
use a warm facecloth, according to Ms. Brown. As
well as increasing circulation, the warmth will help
open up the pores.

Always be gentle when cleansing or touching the
membranes under the eyes, the skin specialist
warns. These membranes are very tender and can
be easily damaged.

• As you get older you should wear less make-up,
Vera Brown says. Since make-up accents wrinkles,
Ms. Brown believes less make-up is more flattering
to an older woman.

• For a good-looking complexion, Vera Brown
recommends a healthful diet. Eliminate coffee,
sugar, salt, fried foods and dairy products for the
best possible skin appearance.

• Smoking increases wrinkles, according to a
study published in the <u>British Medical Journal</u>.
Wrinkles around the eyes and lips, odd colored
complexions, dry skin and leathery skin are more
likely to occur in heavy smokers, the study reports.

• Dr. James Fulton believes that acne and skin problems may be provoked by vitamin supplements and foods that contain iodine. Dr. Fulton works at the Acne Research Institute in Newport Beach, California.

• Psoriasis, acne and poor skin color and appearance are often caused by a diet that is low in the mineral zinc. Zinc is found naturally in liver, seafood, dairy products, meat, eggs and whole-grain products.

• You should protect your skin from overexposure to the sun's ultraviolet rays, to guard against skin cancer and wrinkles.

New research at Cornell University shows that ultraviolet rays actually destroy beta-carotene. Beta-carotene is a natural substance used by the body to create vitamin A. Vitamin A has anti-cancer properties which help prevent lung cancer, bladder cancer and skin cancer. To protect yourself against ultraviolet rays, use a sunscreen with a SPF (sun protection factor) of at least 15 and avoid unnecessary exposure to sunlight.

However, as you protect your skin from the sun's harmful rays, recognize that you may not be getting enough vitamin D. A study in the Journal of Clinical Investigation (10:85) showed that older skin does not produce as much vitamin D from the sun as younger skin does. Vitamin D is important for healthy teeth, bones and muscle tone, and kidney function. Many other vitamins and minerals also need vitamin D to work properly. The sun is the best source of vitamin D, although fish, liver, eggs and fortified milk are also good sources. Eat one of these foods each day to get enough vitamin D. Vitamin D supplements that don't exceed the RDA may also be recommended for people who stay out of the sun.

• Common skin tags may be a warning signal of colon cancer. Skin tags are small flaps of skin, usually occurring in groups in the neck, armpit and groin areas. Researchers at the Mount Sinai School of Medicine in New York have discovered that 86% of their patients with colon polyps, which often become cancerous, also had skin tags. In further testing, 69 percent of their patients with skin tags also had colon polyps. Until now, skin tags were thought to be harmless but cosmetically annoying. If skin tags are annoying, your doctor can remove them. However, the researchers at Mount Sinai suggest that, to be safe, anyone with skin tags should have their stools checked for blood. Since a test for occult (hidden) blood in the stool is a simple and inexpensive procedure, it would be well to be safe and have the test.

• Age spots, the little brown blemishes that often appear later in life, may be helped by pantothenic acid, vitamin B5. A biology professor at Mary Washington College in Virginia, Thomas L. Johnson, Ph.D., claims that daily supplements of pantothenic acid completely cleared age spots in just a few months. However, be careful when considering vitamin B5 supplements. These supplements can change the action of high blood-pressure and blood-thinning drugs. Pantothenic acid may also increase premature skin wrinkles in people who smoke. Pantothenic acid is found naturally in yeast, whole-grain products, liver, salmon, eggs, beans, seeds, peanuts, mushrooms, elderberries and citrus fruit. The best way to prevent age spots is by avoiding exposure to the sun and sunlamps.

• Rough skin on the feet can be a problem. For treatment, soak the feet once a day in warm water. Then gently use a pumice stone to rub away the rough calluses on the feet. Be careful with a pumice stone. You can rub away too much skin, causing bleeding and skin damage. If you soak and rub your feet daily for a couple of weeks, the rough spots should disappear without damaging the feet. Each day after using the pumice stone, apply a good moisturizer or petroleum jelly and cover your feet with socks. Sleeping in the socks will keep the moisturizer on your feet during the night.

• Sudden skin rash could be caused by exposure to high-intensity mercury lamps, according to the

Harvard Medical School Health Letter. High-intensity lamps are usually covered by protective glass to block the ultraviolet rays. However, just a small hole in the protective layer of glass could allow emission of dangerous ultraviolet rays. The New Jersey Department of Health reported a case where 69 out of 89 girls on a school basketball team developed irritation of the eyes and skin rash. The outbreak was caused by a small hole in the protective coating of a mercury vapor light in the gym where the girls' team had just played.

• Photosensitivity is an exaggerated reaction to sunlight, which may be caused by using certain drugs, cosmetics, or perfumes, reports *Patient Care* (6:15). Photosensitivity is not a true allergic reaction, unless the reaction is extremely severe or unusual. Redness, swelling, hives and itching are symptoms of photosensitivity. If your skin is photosensitive, it reacts to the sun more quickly and more severely than normally. Some of the drugs that can lead to photosensitivity are thiazide diuretics, tetracycline, antidiabetics, psoralens, oral contraceptives, antipsychotics, antidepressants, antihistamines, antibacterials, anticancer drugs, and corticosteroids. Coal tar products, coal tar dyes, musk fragrance, some perfumes, and even some sunscreens can also cause photosensitivity.

Smoking — How To Quit The Easy Way And Feel Better

Smoking is known to cause or increase the risks of lung cancer, oral cancer, heart problems, lung diseases, wrinkles, bad breath, the staining of teeth, coated tongue, delayed wound healing and high blood pressure. Within days after you stop smoking, your blood will be able to carry more oxygen. Coughing due to smoke inhalation will be reduced or stop. Your sense of taste and smell will begin to improve.

Many smokers continue smoking even when they realize it is bad for their health because nicotine is very addictive. It is extremely difficult for a smoker to quit smoking because of the physical craving for nicotine which is found in tobacco products.

Smoking is a learned behavior, even though addiction to nicotine makes it hard to quit. Human beings do not have a "need" for the nicotine. The pressures of our peer groups and society have influenced us to smoke. To quit smoking, you must "unlearn" this behavior.

The American Cancer Society, the American Lung Association, Merrell Dow Pharmaceuticals, Seventh Day Adventists and many other organizations have compiled these guidelines to help you "kick the habit".

• The <u>desire</u> to stop smoking will be your biggest

asset when you try to quit. If you don't want to quit, guidelines will not help.

• Examine your reasons for wanting to quit. Besides halting the physical damage of smoking, you may be helping your family and friends, plus saving time and money. Write down at least 10 reasons to quit. Review these reasons daily, and keep adding to the list.

• Decide that you want to quit. Be positive about your decision. Then choose a quitting day and stick to it. If you are a heavy smoker while at work, you may want to quit on a Friday afternoon. By Monday morning, you'll have two smokeless days behind you, and you should be better prepared for the stress of your first smokeless work day.

• Identify the times and feelings you associate with smoking. You may smoke after meals or while you are under stress. When possible, avoid the situations that you associate with smoking. If you feel the desire to smoke every time you have a cup of coffee or an alcoholic drink, cut out the coffee and alcohol as well. Substitute another activity, such as gum chewing or taking a short walk, for the smoking. Learning how to participate in familiar activities without smoking may be the most difficult part of "kicking the habit."

• Organize pleasant and busy activities for the day you will quit. Plan to do things with other people, preferably non-smokers. Keeping an active schedule with plenty of exercise may help you get over the first few days. You may want to have some kind of treat or celebration to start your non-smoking campaign.

• If you are quitting "cold turkey," try to remove all temptations before you start. Throw away all cigarettes. Don't forget the ones you keep at work or in your purse. Remove your ashtrays, lighters and matches.

• Keep your mouth clean. Brush and floss your teeth often so your mouth will taste clean, and you won't have as much urge to smoke. You may want to visit a dental hygienist and have your teeth cleaned within the first few days after you stop smoking. If you schedule the appointment beforehand, this appointment could be one of your first goals as a non-smoker.

• Some people find that sugar-free chewing gum helps you quit smoking by keeping the mouth occupied when you have the urge to pick up a cigarette.

• If you miss having something in your hand to play with, try substituting a pen, pencil or paper clip.

• If you feel the urge to smoke, do something active like taking a bath or shower. Try doing more things with your hands, like writing letters, crafts, sewing, woodwork, housework or yardwork.

• Maintain or improve your physical health. Start regular exercise. Eat healthy meals, including lots of fruit and vegetables. Drink more fluids, including fruit juices and water. Get lots of rest and relaxation. By getting your body in good condition, you will be more able to tolerate the physical symptoms of withdrawal from nicotine. Physical exercise will improve your breathing and blood flow, as well as providing a smoke-free activity.

• Get support. If your spouse smokes, try quitting together. Then, you will be able to support and encourage each other. Try a local stop smoking group in your community. Learning about the hard times other people have experienced while quitting may make your troubles seem smaller. Get involved with people who will support you, and you will improve your chances of staying a non-smoker.

• Remember that smoking is not just a bad habit; smoking also involves an addiction to nicotine. Therefore, you may experience withdrawal symptoms. According to the U.S. Department of Health and Human Services, mood changes, irritability, aggressiveness, anxiety, difficulty in sleeping, drowsiness, weight gain, lower blood pressure, headache, upset stomach and a decrease in the heart rate are common physical reactions to nicotine withdrawal. Usually, the withdrawal symptoms subside within a few days. Since they will end soon, don't let them stop you from achieving a smoke-free life!

• Don't try to have "just one" cigarette, for "old times sake". Just like a drink for a "reformed" alcoholic, one cigarette can begin the smoking cycle again. Even in times of personal crisis, like the death of a loved one or the loss of a job, DON'T succumb to smoking again.

• If you don't quit the first time you try, don't give up. Don't be too hard on yourself. There is a definite physical addiction to nicotine, and it may not be easy to stop. Some people try two or three times before they are able to finally quit. Don't lose faith in God, the ruler of the universe. The one who parted the Red Sea can certainly lead you to victory over a mere weed if you trust and follow Him.

• Not everyone quits "cold turkey", although it's the most successful method of quitting. If you feel that the "cold-turkey" method is not for you, try cutting back on the number of cigarettes, cigars or pipe bowls you smoke each day. Count the number of cigarettes you smoke in an average day, then smoke one less each day. You may need to count out your daily ration every morning. Keep a chart and put away all but the number that you can have each day.

• Congratulate yourself with each step you take as you eliminate smoking. Giving up smoking is hard. Be proud of yourself EACH TIME you pass up smoking a cigarette. According to Merrell Dow Pharmaceuticals Inc., "the risk of smoking again is the highest in the first few months" after you quit. Be careful and reward your achievements. Celebrate your anniversaries of non-smoking. Treat yourself after the first week, the first month and maybe every month after that! You deserve to celebrate!

• Earl Mindell, author of The Vitamin Bible, recommends a variety of nutritional supplements to help overcome the withdrawal from nicotine while trying to stop smoking. Taking one tryptophan tablet, three times daily, seems to help reduce the irritability associated with nicotine withdrawal, he suggests. A good multivitamin, with the vitamin B complex, 100 mg. of cysteine and 300 mg. of vitamin C will help keep the body healthy during the time you are withdrawing from nicotine, says Mindell.

• If you don't want to make the sacrifice to stop smoking now, at least, switch to a low-tar, low-nicotine brand of cigarettes. Be careful not to increase the number of cigarettes you smoke per day. Then, you will be making a small step in the right direction. While you are smoking, Earl Mindell recommends additional vitamins and minerals to help your body cope with the strain that smoking puts on your body. For smokers, Mindell favors a daily multivitamin, with additional amounts of the vitamins C, E and A, and the mineral, selenium.

Snoring
• Rolling a snorer onto his stomach or just changing his position may alleviate the problem. His sleeping on an extra pillow may help.
• If you wear dentures, keep them in all night to avoid snoring, says James Wasco, M.D., in Women's Day magazine (7/29/86). Dentures help keep the mouth in a natural position and may reduce bouts of snoring. Be careful. Some people choke when sleeping with their false teeth.

Sore Throats
• It is important to soothe a sore throat without masking the problem that causes the sore throat. Some over-the-counter medications actually numb the throat. Do not use these products. With the soreness numbed, people tend to talk and work without treating the cause of the sore throat.
• Gargling with salt water is an old home remedy that is still recommended by health professionals. A

professor of internal medicine at the University of Virginia, Dr. Jack Gwaltney, recommends gargling with warm salt water. Dissolve one teaspoon of salt into a small glass of warm water, and gargle every three hours, he suggests. Just <u>gargle</u> with the water. Do not swallow any salt water.

• Drinking a cup of hot tea mixed with honey and lemon juice may ease a sore throat or a coughing spell, but this treatment may also provide food for bacteria to grow in the throat.

Stress — In Adults

Learn to recognize your own body's stress signals. Do you start to snap at people or lose your temper with loved ones? Are you more tired? Do unimportant little things start to bother you? Do you get headaches or body aches? Do you suffer from insomnia? Many of these symptoms can be a sign of personal stress. The first step in alleviating stress is to learn to recognize its signs. Recognizing that you are under stress is necessary before seeking to reduce the stress.

Stress contributes to many physical illnesses, including high blood pressure, colitis, rheumatoid arthritis, ulcers, heart disease and some allergies, according to an article in <u>Women's Day</u> magazine (8/31/85).

Certain events, both good and bad, are known to be stressful. Researchers, Holms and Rahe, have rated several life events by the number of stress points they cause in our lives. Some of these events are planned, but and some are sudden and cannot be anticipated. The top ten life events that cause stress, according to Holms and Rahe, are:

1. Death of a spouse.
2. Divorce.
3. Marital separation.
4. Jail term.
5. Death of a close family member.
6. Personal injury or illness.
7. Marriage.
8. Getting fired from work.
9. Marital reconciliation.
10. Retirement.

• Whenever possible, try not to plan too many high-stress events at the same time. For example, if you buy a home, get married and start a new job all at the same time, you will be under a great deal of stress. However, if you can plan the events so they don't happen together, you can reduce your stress level.

• Your approach to life has a lot to do with how much stress you create for yourself. For example, if you are a perfectionist about your own work and expect others to adhere to your high standards, you are setting yourself up for many stress-filled days. Learning to accept things that are "less than perfect" is important for your health. You don't have to leave your standards completely. If you accept a few "less than perfect" projects, you will lower your stress. Also, remember your strengths and weaknesses. No one can do all things well. Try to improve your strengths and be tolerant of your weaknesses. Don't be too hard on yourself when you discover that you cannot excel at everything. Concentrate your activities where your strengths are.

• Cool your competitive edge. Rather than constantly comparing yourself to others, set your own goals based on your own performance. Don't be constantly trying to get the best parking space, or get ahead of "that car" in traffic. Many times these minor competitions contribute to unnecessary stress in our lives.

• Acknowledge your successes. Celebrate the things you accomplish, no matter how small. If you have a job that is repetitious and if it is difficult to see any progress, create your own accomplishments.

• If you always seem to be concerned with yourself, try reaching out to others. Doing something for someone else may help to put your problems into better perspective. Hopefully, you will become less self-centered as you help the people around you.

• Take time for yourself everyday. Do something that you enjoy. People relax in different ways. Some simply enjoy a few moments of inactivity. Others relax by praying, meditating, reading, exercising, fishing or walking. For a tired mother, it may be spending just a few moments doing something for herself, like working on a craft project, taking the phone off the hook, or taking a bubble bath. Whatever you enjoy, be sure to allow some time for yourself everyday.

• Don't try to bear other people's burdens, unnecessarily. Women in traditional roles are famous for this. The wife and mother often tries to carry the burdens of her husband and children, and she feels very stressed. Learn to recognize that their problems may not be your fault. You can be supportive and loving without carrying burdens that cause stress.

• Beware of traditional holidays or celebrations that were very special to you as a child. Dr. Thomas A. Wehr, a psychiatrist in Washington, D.C. feels that Christmas and other holidays are often the most stress-filled times of our lives. We tend to remember the good times we've had together in the past, remember the loved ones that have died since the last holiday, and feel that nothing can compare to our memories, says Dr. Wehr. Stress is created because of the difference between our past and our present, he explains. To limit the holiday's impact on your stress level, try not to be too sentimental about the past. Concentrate on making the current holiday memorable.

• Don't be afraid to get help. Asking for help is not a sign of weakness, but rather a sign that you know your own limitations. Many people are afraid to ask for help, and then the stress of the burdens they are carrying becomes overwhelming. But asking for help, to complete a project, ease the burden of housework or to talk to a professional counselor, is a positive way of coping with stress.

• Don't be afraid to cry. Research has shown that crying is a natural and healthy way to deal with stress. Crying helps focus your emotions and provides a release. For crying to be most helpful, though, it must be done in private. You should be comfortable and be able to cry as long as you'd like. If you cry in front of a business associate or someone you don't want to see you cry, you may feel so guilty about crying that it won't relieve your stress. Try not always to hold back your tears.

• Music is now being recognized and used by professional therapists to help relieve and treat stress. According to Alicia Gibbons, Ph.D., the past president of the National Association for

Music Therapy, music can change the breathing rate, the heart rate, and the level of stress someone is experiencing. Dr. Gibbons suggests that whatever music you prefer, the music that causes you to relax will be most helpful. Songs from your past that you associate with good times can bring back those good feelings. However, the therapist prefers music without lyrics so you don't get caught up in listening to words. After having a stressful experience, lying down with your eyes closed and listening to the music should alleviate some of the symptoms of stress.

After a few sessions of using the same music as relaxation therapy, your body becomes trained to relax whenever you hear that music. For example, a person had been using one aerobics tape for several months. The audio tape included several different segments, ending with a calm time of deep breathing. One day in the midst of something else, the person heard the song that was used during the cool-down. Immediately, she felt peaceful and relaxed. Yet, it took her several minutes to realize why she knew the song. After many hours of relaxing to that music, she subconsciously associated it with peace and serenity.

Music can also help prepare a person for a stressful situation. If someone dreads going to a dentist or has an important business meeting, they can play their "calming" music on the way there. The right music will help you approach stressful events in a calm and serene manner.

If you have a stressful job, try to avoid bringing stress home to your family. Taking your frustrations out on your family and friends may add to their stress, says Dr. Barbara Mackoff. There should be a time for discussing your problems with your family, and your family should be able to support you. But learn the difference between having their support and making them share the burden of your stress. Mackoff, who wrote <u>Leaving The Office Behind</u>, gives some practical suggestions:

• Change clothes when you come home from work. This may be the opposite of the "dress for success" model but it is important because it is a way to leave the job behind.

• Exercise, on your way home after work or as soon as you get home, can give you a chance to clear your mind as well as rejuvenate your body. Regular exercise will help improve your circulation, lower your blood pressure, and allow you to cope better with the stresses you face.

• Have a goodbye ritual as you leave your workplace. If you can lock up, clean up or finish up in the same way each day, it helps you to say "goodbye" to your job. Having a farewell ritual will start moving your focus from work to your family.

• As you are leaving work, think about your family. Picture your spouse and children. Center your thoughts on them, their day's activities, and how much you miss them. This will help you shift your mind from work to your family and help leave your job stress behind.

• If possible, relax on your way home. If you must think through some work-related problems, do it before you get home. Resolve everything about your job before you get home if possible. Then, when you get home, you can concentrate on your family.

• If you are still stressed when you arrive home, greet everyone and then take a few quiet minutes for yourself. While you are alone, close your eyes, take some deep breaths, and work through your frustrations. If you yell when you are under pressure, yell into a pillow or in the shower or have an imaginary conversation with the work associate who is bothering you. Then, leave your problems and spend time with your family.

Stress — In Children

Handling stress in children can be a very delicate, but important, concern for parents. While in the first grade, a child developed a severe case of hives.

After several months of treatment by a dermatologist, another doctor suggested that the hives were a result of stress. The child's parents were shocked. Eventually, they discovered that she was afraid of her first-grade teacher. She loved school, but feared her teacher. That June when the school year ended, so did the hives, and they never returned.

As adults, we sometimes feel that children's problems are not very serious and that children do not feel stress. However, problems we may consider to be minor, might be extremely stressful for a child. Here are some suggestions for helping to cope with stress in children, most of which are recommended by Loraine Stern, M.D. in Woman's Day magazine (7/29/86).

• Whenever possible, prepare your child for upcoming events that can be stressful. For example, discussing a new baby in the family, a trip to the hospital, doctor or dentist, and starting school or preschool. If the child understands about the coming event and is able to ask questions and get answers, the event will not cause as much stress.

• Be very supportive. If a child is feeling stress, your support and encouragement are very important.

• Accept that your child is under stress. Be sure to treat the child's problem as a real and important situation. Don't demean the child or pass off the problem as something every child must go through. Even a dark room at night can cause great stress if a child is frightened by the dark.

• Share a quiet time with your child every day. Quiet, quality time with each child will allow him to share concerns with you.

• Watch for the physical signs of stress in your child. Children, more than adults, may have a difficult time expressing their concerns. Headaches, unusual irritability, hives, abdominal pain and tiredness may be stress-related. A quick change in actions or habits, like suddenly disliking school, uncharacteristic misbehavior, or losing friends, may also be signs of stress.

• Don't let your child hear fearful expressions of concerns about life or the future. Present a strong faith to your child that God is in charge and that all is well, while not denying real problems such as death or injury.

• Don't place your burdens on your children. Children often know when their parents are under stress, so be calm before trying to help your child.

• If your child is under extreme stress, help is available. Professional counselors, including therapists, guidance counselors and ministers, can help. It is better to help the child when problems occur, than to let him suffer from anxiety for many years.

Stroke Prevention

Strokes are the third leading cause of death in the United States. However, with proper care, you can reduce your risk of having a stroke. Diabetics, smokers, blacks, men, people with a family or personal history of heart disease or strokes, women taking oral contraceptives, and those over age 60 are at high risk of having a stroke.

To reduce your risk of stroke:

• Stop smoking.

• Control your blood pressure. Have your blood pressure monitored regularly, and keep it below 140/90. Limit your intake of salt, including salt-cured foods, especially if you are black. Many people, including almost all blacks have a "salt conservation gene" that makes them retain salt and water and have high blood pressure. The only way to combat this tendency is with a diet that is almost salt-free — less than one gram per day from all sources.

• Lose weight.

• Learn to manage your stress.

• Get regular exercise.

• Avoid alcohol. Alcohol raises blood pressure and counteracts the effects of exercise, a study from the Medical College of Wisconsin reports.

• Do not use illegal drugs. Use of cocaine, heroin and amphetamines has been liked to an increased risk of stroke.

• Eat well. Your diet should consist of low-cholesterol, low-fat foods.

Also see: **Cholesterol Build-Up**.

• Keep diabetes in control. High blood sugar levels in diabetics increase the possibility of having a stroke.

Report any of the following early warning signs of stroke to your doctor immediately. Quick medical treatment may help prevent a more serious stroke from happening. Here are some of the signs of having a small stroke, as identified by the American Heart Association:

• Change in vision, such as a sudden loss of sight or double vision.

• Difficulty with speech.

• Unexplained headaches or dizziness.

• Impaired judgment.

• Numbness, weakness or tingling sensations.

• Sudden change in mental abilities.

• Sudden change in personality.

• Any symptoms that seem to occur only on one side of the body.

Styes
Styes are small pimples that form on the outer eyelid or just inside the eyelid. Most styes appear

only for a few days, then disappear without any treatment.

To help heal a sty at home, put a hot cloth directly on the sty for about 10 minutes, four times daily, suggests The Merck Manual. Do not pop the white section of the sty. If a sty with a whitehead appears at the base of an eyelash, you may pull out the eyelash. Removing the eyelash will safely break the sty and start the healing process. If a sty becomes unusually large, or if it is growing on the inside of the eyelid, have it checked by a doctor. An antibiotic may be required, either one prescribed by your doctor or an over-the-counter ointment that you can buy without prescription.

Temporomandibular Joint (TMJ) Syndrome

Many dentists and orthodontists are now specializing in treating temporomandibular joint (TMJ) syndrome. TMJ syndrome occurs when the muscles that control the jaw joints go into spasms. These muscles are related to facial, back and neck muscles so the spasms can cause severe headaches, earaches, and pain throughout the head, neck and arms.

Many things can cause TMJ syndrome:

• Sometimes getting hit on the head or being in a car accident can knock the jaw "out of joint."

• Other times it can be caused by an imbalance in the structure of the jaws at birth. With an imbalance, the features on one side of the face may be higher than those on the other side.

• Many times the syndrome is caused by people grinding their teeth and tensing their jaw muscles as they react to stress.

To relieve the TMJ pain, which may occur in the neck, arms, or face, try one or more of the following:

• Have a dentist or orthodontist fit you with a small plastic appliance that is worn in the mouth. This appliance will help put the jaw back into its correct position over several months and reduce the stress on the TMJ muscles. Orthodontic appliances and surgery are the only ways to actually fix the TMJ problem permanently. An appliance or surgery will actually move the jaw into its correct position and eliminate the problem. Wearing the appliance rather than resorting to surgery is all that's required in most cases.

• Apply heat to the jaw area. Hot cloths, a heating pad or a heating ointment may provide some relief.

• Apply cold to the jaw area. Some people respond better to cold treatments.

• Massage the muscles. A good massage of the jaw muscles, the neck and the back may help reduce pain.

• Practice stress reduction and relaxation techniques. Become conscious of how your body reacts to stress. If you are grinding your teeth in your sleep at night, you may be causing TMJ problems. Some people tense the muscles in the jaw when they are straining to move an object, opening something, or during a bowel movement. Teach yourself not to tighten your jaw muscles while straining.

Thumb Sucking

Thumb sucking starts out as a natural "soother" for a baby or young child. However, any children who continue to suck on their fingers or thumbs after the age of four can cause permanent damage to their teeth, gums, and the shape of their mouths. Many times braces or other orthodontic appliances are needed because a child has continued to suck his fingers or thumbs past four years of age.

The best methods for breaking thumb sucking are those which involve both the parents and the child. The problem should be discussed with the child, explaining why it is time to stop this habit. Positive reinforcement, such as giving the child a small reward for every day without sucking, is a good start. However, positive reinforcement does not work with all children.

Another suggestion is to coat the fingers or thumb

with an unpleasant-tasting substance. You can buy alum or special formulas, available over-the-counter at drugstores, that are made specifically for children with thumb-sucking problems. Some of these commercial preparations are hard to lick off and so unpleasant tasting that they often break thumb sucking in just a few days, according to <u>Pediatrics</u> (78·1).

Tooth Decay   See: **Dental Problems**

Weight Loss
   Eat fewer calories and exercise. These are two very simple rules that can contribute to safe, gradual weight-loss. However, most Americans seem to want a "pill" that they can take so they will be thinner "overnight". For many people, losing weight means a lifelong commitment to proper nutrition and regular exercise. This may be a drastic change from a sedentary lifestyle and the food that most of us eat.
   Exercise alone does not cause weight to "just disappear." But it usually will perk up your metabolism and your rate of burning calories — even in the hours after your exercise. Exercise sometimes actually depresses appetite. If you

exercise and don't eat more, you <u>will</u> lose weight.

Since the most important element of exercising is actually "doing it," it is important that the exercise you choose be something you will continue. Most people who are sedentary find it difficult to stick to an exercise program. According to the Federal Trade Commission, 70% of the people who join a fitness club or health spa will quit within just three months.

According to <u>Editorial</u> <u>Research</u> <u>Reports</u>, exercising also helps combat some other problems associated with being overweight. Even if exercising doesn't cause weight loss, it can lower high blood pressure, increase one's self-esteem and reduce depression. Therefore, exercise is worthwhile, even without actual weight loss, <u>Editorial</u> <u>Research</u> <u>Reports</u> says.

Exercise also helps some people lose weight because it increases their awareness of their bodies. Many people who start an exercise program are suddenly aware of what and how much they are eating. Exercising, and feeling those tired muscles, can be a good reminder to people that they are trying to lose weight.

<u>Consumer</u> <u>Guide</u> has listed some guiding principles that will help people choose a form of exercise that they will enjoy and continue to participate in:

• Time. You must choose an activity that you are willing to devote time to every day or every other day. Downhill skiing may be something you enjoy, but if you can participate for only one day a week, during three months of the year, you will need another form of exercise as well.

• Pleasure. The exercise you choose must be something you enjoy doing. Be willing to try several different activities at first so you don't limit yourself to what you have tried before. You may discover that a form of exercise you thought would be boring is perfectly suited to your needs and enjoyment.

• Variety. Choose a variety of activities that you enjoy. You may discover that aerobics classes during the week and a long walk or hike on the weekend are a perfect combination for you.

• Success. Don't undermine your exercise by feeling guilty if you miss your planned activity. Look forward to your next time of exercise. Celebrate the successes you have enjoyed during your exercising. If you get discouraged while increasing the length or intensity of your exercise, try going back briefly to the same routine or amount of exercise as when you first started your program.. You will find that it seems easy compared to what you can do after building up your endurance through regular exercise.

• Spouse. If you are married, having the support of your spouse can be very important. Finding an activity that you can do together can be great. Even if your spouse can't or won't participate with you, moral support will make it easier for you to continue with regular exercise.

• Groups. Many people find that the support of a group makes regular exercise easier to continue. This doesn't mean you have to join an expensive fitness club or take a class. Just getting together with a small group of friends who are willing to meet regularly and go for a walk can help. The companionship of friends, knowing you are not alone, and enjoying exercise as a social activity are very helpful.

• Money. Some people find that paying for an exercise class is the best incentive for them to continue exercising. You may feel a strong urge to attend all the classes because you don't want to "waste the money." If this works for you, keep paying for classes in advance!

Don't let your children get overweight. According to research published in the journal, <u>Pediatrics</u> (6:80), babies and children who are overweight will have an increased tendency to become overweight adults. If one or both of a child's parents are overweight, that also increases the child's chances of becoming an overweight adult.

The attitudes of parents toward eating will influence how much the child eats. The old saying, "Eat to live, don't live to eat" is very appropriate. Don't pile on food and urge children to "clean their plates"

Try not to use food as a reward. For children with a tendency to gain weight, getting dessert if they finish all their dinner is not a good idea. Children should be taught that food is important to their health and necessary for their bodies. They should not be taught that sweets are the only "good" food or that sweet drinks are the best drinks.

Moderation is the key. Parents should try to promote a "healthy" weight for their children rather than promoting extreme thinness. This should help the child and the parents accept each other as they are, yet yearn for the healthiest weight, diet and lifestyle.

Use less caloric foods for children who are overweight. If the child is over two years of age, use skim milk. Until the age of two, the extra fat in the whole milk is helpful for proper development of the brain. Limit sweets and soft drinks. Drink more water Reduce the amount of fried foods in the diet. Remove the skin from chicken and trim the fat from red meat. If you don't mention the word "diet" the child probably will not notice these changes.

Exercise may be the easiest way for overweight children to lose weight. According to an article in <u>Woman's Day</u> magazine (11/11/86), the more hours a child watches TV each day, the greater the chance of that child being overweight. Simply turning off the TV and telling a child to go outside and play can do wonders for the child's waistline. Children who exercise with their parents have the most success with weight loss. The parent' influence cannot be emphasized enough. Parents need to set an example and be willing to help children lose weight.

A Final Word

The health tips in this book are based on reports of common sense, natural healing methods, but don't overlook the supernatural healing power of God. God is out Creator and the Master Physician. God sent His only Son, Jesus Christ, into this world to give us everlasting life. Jesus worked miracles 2,000 years ago. God still works miracles today. If you put your faith in God, by following Jesus Christ, the Bible promises that your prayers will be answered according to God's will.

If you would like to know more about how to know God and have eternal life through a personal relationship with Jesus Christ, please write to: FC&A, Dept. JC 87, 103 Clover Green, Peachtree City, Georgia, 30269. We believe getting to know God better will change your life!

May the blessings of God, the Father, Son and Holy Spirit be with you as you search for a healthy life on earth and seek Him for everlasting life.

Appendix One — Special Agencies To Consult

This is just a small list of the many agencies that are able to give you health information. For other toll-free numbers, call your long distance information operator at 1-800-555-1212 and ask if a specific agency has a toll-free number.

Acne Hotline (800) 235-ACNE
(in CA 800-225-ACNE)
Information on how to treat and prevent acne.

Aging Hotline (414) 272-4130
Information from the National Geriatrics Society.

Aging Information (301) 496-1752
Information from the National Institute on Aging.

AIDS Hotline (800) 342-2437
How to prevent AIDS and care for AIDS victims.

Alzheimer's and Related Diseases Information (612) 679-4016
Information from the Association for Alzheimer's and Related Diseases. Specializes in counselling and supporting families of people suffering

from Alzheimer's.

Arthritis Foundation   (404) 872-7100
Information from the Arthritis Foundation.
Mailing address: 1314 Spring Street, N.W.
Atlanta, Georgia 30309.

Arthritis Information (800) 327-3027
Information from the Arthritis Medical Center

Asthma-Allergy Hotline (800) 558-1035
(in Wisconsin call collect to 414-272-1004)
Information from the American Academy of
Allergy and Immunology

The Asthma and Allergy Foundation
(202) 293-2950
1302 18th Street N.W. — Suite 303, Washington,
D.C.   20036. Write for a complete list of the
products that are truly non-allergenic.

Asthma Hotline   (800) 222-LUNG
Information from the National Asthma Center at
the National Jewish Hospital.

Biofeedback Information
(303) 422-8436
Information from the Biofeedback Society of

America, 4301 Owens Street, Wheat Ridge, Colorado 80033. Bio-feed back is a natural way to learn self-control over the body.

Birth Defects Hotline (800) 24-CLEFT
(in Pa. 800-23-CLEFT)
Information for parents of children with birth defects, sponsored by the American Cleft Palate Educational Foundation. Will help refer parents to local specialists and support groups.

Blindness Information (800) 221-3004
Information from the National Society to Prevent Blindness.

Cancer Hotline (800) 4-CANCER
(in New York City 212-794-7982; in Washington, D.C. 202-636-5700; Alaska 800-638-6070; or in Hawaii 808-524-1234)
Information from the National Cancer Institute, P.O. Box K, Bethesda, Maryland, 20814.

Diabetes Information (800) 327-3027
Information from the American Diabetes Association.

Eye Care Helpline (800) 222-EYES
(8 a.m.-5 p.m. all time zones) Information from

the Foundation of the American Academy of Ophthalmology. Will refer people over 65 years of age to a local ophthalmologist.

Health Information (800) 336-4797
(in Va. 703-522-2590)
Information from the National Health Information Clearinghouse of the Office of Disease Prevention and Health Promotion. Answers questions about where to call or write for health information on a specific topic.

Hearing Information (800) 638-8255
Information from the National Association for Hearing and Speech Action.

Hearing Screening Test (800) 222-EARS
Use a telephone with good reception and this number gives you access to a two-minute hearing test. Local facilities are recommended if you seem to have hearing problems.

Heart Hotline (800) 241-6993
(in Ga. 404-523-0826; collect) Information from the Association of Heart Patients, Inc. on heart disease.

Heart Information
Information from the American Heart Association, 7320 Greensville Avenue, Dalla, Texas 75231.

Impotence Hotline (800) 221-5517
(9 a.m.-5 p.m. M-F Pacific Time) Information from the Impotence Foundation is available to men and women.

Impotence Information (800) 843-4315
Information from the Impotence Information Center, Dept USA, P.O. Box 9, Minneapolis, MN 55440.

Liver Information (201) 857-2626
Information about diseases of the liver, gall bladder and bile ducts from the American Liver Foundation, 998 Pompton Avenue, Cedar Grove, New Jersey 07009.

Mental Health Information (800) 344-8795
(in Va. 800-468-1359) A series of taped information on mental health called The Headline. Sponsored by Saint Albans Psychiatric Hospital in Radford, Virginia. Over 125 topics accessible only by touch-tone phone.

Organ Donor Hotline (800) 24-DONOR
  (in Va. 1-800-552-2138)
  Information on how to donate the life-saving gift
of your organs.

Pacemaker Information (414) 659-0919
  Information from the International Association of
Pacemaker Patients.

Poisoning Information Hotline
  (412) 681-6669 (open 24 hours)
  Call if someone has swallowed poision or something you think MAY be poisonous.

Premenstrual Syndrome (PMS) Information
  (800) 222-4PMS
  Information from PMS Access. Or you can write
directly to: PMS Access, Box 9326, Madison,
Wisconsin, 53715.

Second Surgical Opinion Hotline
  (800) 638-6833
  (or in Maryland 800-492-6603)
  Information on surgeons in your area who are
willing to be consulted for second opinions regarding surgery.

Sodium Information (800) 622-DASH
Information on sodium content of any food, from the Mrs. Dash Company.

Stroke and Stroke Prevention (800) 638-8255
Write to: National Institute of Neurological and Communicative Disorder and Stroke, Office of Scientific and Health Reports, Bldg. 31, Room 8A06, Bethesda, Maryland 20892.

Tinnitus Information (503) 248-9985
Information from the American Tinnitus Association on ear noises and "ringing in the ears."

Tourette Syndrome (800) 237-0717
Information on Tourette Syndrome. Call toll-free or write: Tourette Syndrome, 42-40 Bell Blvd., Bayside, New York 11361.

Appendix Two — Bibliography

Arthritis Foundation. *Overcoming Rheumatoid Arthritis: What You Can Do For Yourself.* Arthritis Foundation. Atlanta, Georgia. 1983.

Berkow, M.D. Editor-in-Chief. *The Merck Manual.* Merck Sharp & Dohme Research Laboratories. Rahway, New Jersey. 1982.

Cawood, Frank W. *Vitamin Side Effects Revealed.* FC&A Publishing. Peachtree City, Georgia. 1986.

Cawood, Frank W. and Janice McCall Failes. *Allergies Relieved Naturally.* FC&A Publishing. Peachtree City, Georgia. 1985.

Cawood, Frank W. and Janice McCall Failes. *Hidden Health Secrets.* FC&A Publishing. Peachtree City, Georgia. 1986.

Cawood, Frank W., Rita Warmack, Janice McCall Failes and Gayle R. Cawood. *Arteries Cleaned Out Naturally: Scientific Facts and Fancies.* FC&A Publishing. Peachtree City, Georgia. 1986.

Cawood, Gayle, M.Ed., Janice McCall Failes and Frank W. Cawood. *Prescription Drug*

Encyclopedia. FC&A Publishing. Peachtree City, Georgia. 1986.

Ellis, Jeffrey W., M.D. and Editors of Consumer Guide®. *Medical Symptoms and Treatments.* Publications International. Skokie, Illinois. 1983.

Failes, Janice McCall and Frank W. Cawood. *Natural Healing Encyclopedia.* FC&A Publishing. Peachtree City, Georgia. 1987.

Frank, Martha Ross. *The American Medical Association's Handbook of First Aid and Emergency Care.* Random House. New York, New York. 1980.

Gelb, Harold, D.M.D. and Paula M. Siegel. *Killing Pain Without Prescription.* Harper and Row. New York, New York. 1980.

Gimlin, Hoyt, editor. *Staying Healthy: Nutrition, Lifestyle and Medicine.* Editorial Research Reports. Congressional Quarterly Inc. Washington, D.C. 1984.

Hopkins, Harold. "The Dental Plaque Battle is Endless But Worth It". *FDA Consumer.* Vol 18. No. 7. September 1984.

Johnson, G. Timothy, M.D. and Stephen E. Gold-
finger, M.D., editors. *The Harvard Medical School
Health Letter Book.* Harvard University Press.
Cambridge, Massachusetts. 1981.

Kepler, James. *How To Get A Good Night's Sleep.*
Budlong Press Company. Chicago, Illinois. 1980.

Kurland, Howard D., M.D. *Quick Headache Relief
without Drugs.* William Morrow and Company,
Inc. New York, New York. 1977.

Mindell, Earl and Hester Mundis. *The Vitamin
Bible.* Warner Books, Inc. New York, New York.
1985.

National Enquirer. *Living With Arthritis.* Pocket
Books. New York, New York. 1985.

Rumsey, Timothy, M.D. and Orlo Otteson *A Physician's Complete Guide to Medical Self-Care.*
Rutledge Press. New York, New York. 1981.

"Quitting". An educational brochure regarding
smoking. Merrell Dow Pharmaceuticals, Inc. Cin-
cinnati, Ohio. 1984.

Steincrohn, Peter J. M.D,. F.A.C.P. *How To Be*

Lazy, Healthy and Fit. Funk & Wagnalls. New York, New York. 1968.

"Why People Smoke Cigarettes". U.S. Department of Health and Human Services. Rockville, Maryland. 1983.

"HE DIED WITH ARTERIES LIKE A BABY"

Clean Artery

Artery 50% clogged by fat and cholesterol

Artery 90% clogged by fat and cholesterol

(By Frank K. Wood)

Can your arteries be cleaned out naturally? That's what many doctors are wondering after an autopsy of a famous nutrition expert.

The "free from artery disease" theory of the nutrition expert may be proven by his death! The doctor who performed the autopsy was, in his own words, "amazed to find no evidence of coronary artery disease in a man of his age (69)". He said that the nutrition expert died with "arteries like a baby". What's even more amazing is that the nutrition expert was diagnosed as actually having coronary artery disease 30 years earlier when he was 39 years old.

Case studies like the well–known nutritionist's may be atypical. Now, a new book, *"Arteries Cleaned Out Naturally"* contains information on a natural, drug free way to stop heart and artery disease.

LIFE SAVING SECRETS REVEALED IN THIS NEW BOOK

- How to tell if you're having a heart attack...or just indigestion.
- A new treatment that opens up arteries without surgery.
- Amazing, easy ways to keep your arteries clean.
- A simple step that can help 1/3 of all Americans avoid a heart attack.
- Why foot problems are associated with high rates of heart attack.
- Exercise. . . one type that's very harmful . . . another type that can help.
- Definitions of terms like coronary thrombosis, aneurysm, angina, etc.
- The amazing story of HDL's. The body's natural system that helps keep the arteries clean.
- How to add 10 years to your life.
- The truth about cholesterol and hardening of the arteries.

"DO YOU KNOW THESE LITTLE KNOWN NATURAL HEALTH TIPS AND CURES?"

AN AMAZING TREASURE TROVE OF 217 CURES AND HEALTH TIPS

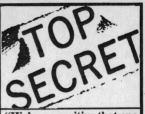

(By Frank K. Wood)

FC&A, a Peachtree City, Georgia, publisher, announced today the release of a new book for the general public, *"Natural Healing Encyclopedia"*.

LOOK AT SOME OF THE SECRETS REVEALED IN THIS NEW BOOK

- Alzheimer's Disease from your cookware? Check your pots.
- Lose weight without eating less. When you eat can help you lose weight.
- Inner ear noises could be from a lack of these vitamins in your diet.
- High blood pressure? Natural, drug-free ways to bring it down.
- Feeling tired? This simple remedy helps.
- See how a tennis ball can keep your mate from snoring.
- A quick fix for canker sores.
- Hangover? The U.S. Government's remedy.
- PMS relief.
- How being "lady-like" can cause this disease.
- Pet therapy for people.

- 2 minerals that can help many diabetics.
- A Q-tip® may actually help get rid of hiccups.
- Ways to keep calm when feeling stressed.
- A nutritional supplement helps poor memory.
- Back pain? A $10 piece of wood can end it.
- Vitamins and minerals that may slow down aging.
- Wrinkles are unavoidable, right? Wrong!
- Strokes are totally unrelated to heart disease. Right? Wrong.
- Kidney stones? This helps.
- Sleeplessness. Causes and common-sense remedies.
- Learn how a cobweb can help when you get a cut in the woods.
- Eat this and cut in half your chances of getting certain cancers.
- Breast disease? Here's a vitamin that shrinks most non-cancerous lumps?
- How to get rid of corns and calluses — for good.
- Allergy and asthma sufferers: This vitamin can help many.
- Got a bad cough? Take this common beverage.

- Arthritis? There's nothing "fishy" about this treatment from the deep, blue sea.
- Take this and lower cholesterol.
- Help for gallstones.

IT'S EASY TO ORDER

Just return this notice with your name and address and a check for **$11.97** plus $3.00 shipping to our address: **FC&A, Dept. SHZ-8**, 103 Clover Green, Peachtree City, Georgia 30269. We will send you a copy of *"Natural Healing Encyclopedia"* right away.

Save! Return this notice with **$23.94** + $3.00 for two books. (No extra shipping.)

Satisfaction guaranteed or your money back.

You must cut out and return this notice with your order. Copies not accepted!

IMPORTANT — FREE GIFT OFFER

All orders will receive a free gift. Order right away!

©FC&A 1988

"PRESCRIPTION DRUG KILLS DOCTOR"

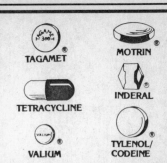

(By Frank K. Wood)

An Atlanta doctor has died from a freak drug reaction on a trip overseas. An infection he had didn't clear up after taking a drug so he took a different drug, too. The two drugs reacted with each other and caused crystallization in his kidneys. He had kidney failure and died a few days later.

WHAT YOUR DOCTOR DOESN'T TELL YOU ABOUT THE SIDE EFFECTS OF PRESCRIPTION DRUGS

This tragedy points to the fact that most doctors don't tell their patients about the side effects of the drugs they prescribe.

The reaction that killed the doctor and many other prescription drug side effects are clearly described in a new book, *"Prescription Drug Encyclopedia"*.

THE GOOD EFFECTS OF PRESCRIPTION DRUGS

We all take drugs prescribed by our doctor for their good effects, like relieving pain, fighting infection, birth control, aiding sleep, calming down, fighting coughs, colds or allergies, or lowering heartbeat and blood pressure.

DO YOU HAVE ANY OF THESE BAD SIDE EFFECTS?

Prescription drugs can cause headache, upset stomach, constipation, stuffy nose, short breath, high blood pressure, fear and ringing sounds.

LATEST FACTS ON EACH DRUG

The book describes more than 400 of the most-often-used drugs. Facts are given in easy-to-understand words.

EASY TO READ

The book lists brand names, money-saving generic names, good effects, side effects, and warnings.

It explains drug categories. (For example: a drug may be called an "analgesic" . . . analgesic means "pain reliever").

Order this 30,000 word, easy-to-understand book explaining more than 400 drugs, edited by two pharmacists, right away.

IT'S EASY TO ORDER

Just return this notice with your name and address and a check for **$11.97** plus $3.00 shipping to our following address: **FC&A, Dept. PHZ-8,** 103 Clover Green, Peachtree City, Georgia, 30269. We will send you a copy of *"Prescription Drug Encyclopedia"* right away.

Save! Return this notice with **$23.94 + $3.00** for two books. (No extra shipping.)

Satisfaction guaranteed or your money back.

You must cut out and return this notice with your order. Copies will not be accepted!

IMPORTANT — FREE GIFT OFFER EXPIRES IN 30 DAYS

All orders mailed in 30 days will receive a free gift. Order right away!

©FC&A 1988

"DO YOU KNOW THESE TOP SECRET WAYS TO DEFEAT OLD AGE?"

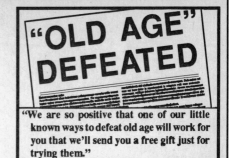

(By Frank K. Wood)

FC&A, a Peachtree City, Georgia, health publisher, announced today the release of a new book for the general public, *"Encyclopedia of Top Secret Ways to Defeat Old Age"*.

LOOK AT SOME OF THE LITTLE KNOWN WAYS TO DEFEAT OLD AGE REVEALED IN THIS NEW BOOK

- Senile? Don't bet on it. This little known secret can restore the mind in many people.
- Alzheimer's Disease from the air you breathe? Read this.
- Chest pain is directly related to heart disease severity. Right? Not always.
- Causes and common-sense remedies for sleeplessness and feeling tired.
- Arthritis? There's nothing "fishy" about this treatment from the deep, blue sea.
- Looking older? "Aging symp-toms" may only be a side effect of a prescription drug you're taking.
- Poor hearing could be from a lack of these vitamins in your diet.
- A nutritional supplement to help poor memory.

HOW MOTHER NATURE CAN HELP DEFEAT FATHER TIME

- Age spots? Apply this fruit juice, and they disappear.
- Breast disease? Here's a vitamin that makes most non-cancerous lumps go away.
- Take this and lower cholesterol.
- Cold sensitive? Take this vitamin.
- Constipated? Drink this.
- 2 minerals that can help many diabetics.
- Help for gallstones.
- Pain? This blocks it.
- Ulcers-stop them from returning.
- How to prevent varicose veins.

THESE WORK AT ANY AGE

- This vitamin helps your body heal.
- Help for your complexion.
- Back problems? Do this to avoid unnecessary muscle strain.
- Makeup wearers - less makeup can make you more attractive.
- Some drug combinations can kill

IT'S EASY TO ORDER

Just return this notice with your name and address and a check for **$11.97** plus $3.00 handling to our address: **FC&A, Dept. OHZ-8**, 103 Clover Green, Peachtree City, Georgia 30269. We will send you a copy of *"Encyclopedia of Top Secret Ways to Defeat Old Age"* right away.

Save! Return this notice with **$23.94 + $3.00** for two books. (No extra shipping.)

You get a no-time-limit guarantee of satisfaction or your money back.

You must cut out and return this notice with your order. Copies will not be accepted!

IMPORTANT — FREE GIFT OFFER

All orders will receive a free gift. Order right away.

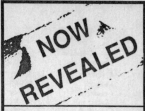